LONGEVITY AND LIFE CYCLE SAVINGS

How to live well to 100 years old

INTRODUCTION

Everybody deserves a long and healthy life. Since there is life on this planet, people on earth struggle to know the facts of death and age. But the truth of mortality did not come to their notice, but to some degree, they managed to control the degenerative effects of the aging process.

Longevity is a term generally referred to as' long life' or' significant lifespan.' The word ' longevity' is sometimes used as a synonym for statistical' life expectancy.' Various factors contribute to the longevity of an organism. Longevity can also be sought by those who do not want eternal life to experience more of life or make a greater contribution to humanity. You will help make medication for longevity and happier, safer lives a reality.

Fear of death makes longevity more desirable than the love of life; I think. Large amounts are expended on intervention in medical systems that support life on the edge of life. In some cases, this is done because of the quality of life. What does current research say about longevity improvements and the

impacts of longer life on the quality of life?

CHAPTER ONE

Meaning of Human Nature

What kind of animal is the human being? A smart, talkative, upright ape with love for material possessions is the obvious answer. But what about the more complex human nature concept? This is more complicated. Basically speaking, are people good or bad? It is a question that has been asked endlessly in all of humanity. Philosophers have been debating for thousands of years whether we have an essentially good nature that is manipulated by society or whether we have an evil nature that is regulated by society. Psychology has provided some facts that could transform the old debate.

One thing to ask about our most essential features is to glance at children. The minds of babies are a wonderful example of human nature. Babies are people with the absolute minimum cultural influence-they have not many friends, they've never been to school. We You cannot even control your own bowels, yet alone chat their language so that their mind is as naïve as a human mind could get.

The only drawback is that it is difficult to measure their views because of the lack of language. We usually ask people to participate in tests, give them directions, or ask them to answer the questions, which both require language. Baby might be cuter to deal with, but their obedience isn't known to them. What's an interesting psychologist to do?

Luckily, to express your views, you do not actually have to speak. Babies reach out to things that they want or want and tend to look for things that interest them longer. Such tests were used by groundbreaking researchers at Yale University in the US to test babies ' minds. Our results suggest that even the youngest people have an instinct to choose good rather than bad.

How can the tests say that? Imagine you're a child. As you have a short period of time, the test is simpler and more engaging than most psychological experiments. The scene of a sparkling green hill, the puppets are cut-off shapes with a wobbly a triangle, eye stick, a circle and a square, each in its own brights. It was a kind of puppet show. What appeared next is a short play when one of the forms tried to climb the hill, fight back and fall down again. Then the two other types got involved, either by supporting the hill climber, by pushing up from behind, or by pushing the climber down from above.

There's already something fantastic, emotionally, here. All humans should view the events in the play. The marionettes are just types. You don't make human sounds or display human emotions. They just pass, but everyone reads these gestures purposefully and exposes their characters. You may argue that this "mind-reading," even in children, shows that believing in other minds is part of our human nature.

Which happened next teaches us even more about human nature. Great expectations. After the show, kids were given a choice to reach either the aid or the obstacle shape, and it turned out that they could reach the helper much more. This

9

can be explained if you read the events in relation to motivations-the forms don't move just randomly, but they have shown that the shape that pushes up "will help out" (and so is nice), and the shape that pushes down "will cause problems" (and so is unpleasant).

Such findings were also verified by the researchers. Kids saw a second scene in which the outline of the climber chose to move either towards the aid shape or the obstructive type. In each of the two cases, the time children spent looking showed what they felt about the test. When the climber went to the challenge, the babies appeared even longer than the climber moved to the assistant.

It made sense when the babies were shocked when the climber came to the obstacle. The happy ending would be going towards the aid form, and it was clear what the child planned. If the climber went towards the barrier, it was surprising to see someone kissing him as much as you or I would be shocked.

The way to make sense of this finding is if kids have assumptions about how people would work through their pre-cultural brains. We not only view motivation as the motion of forms but prefer motivation rather than challenge motivation.

This does not resolve the human nature question. A cynic would argue that it demonstrates only that children have an interest in themselves and expect others to be the same. But at least it shows that the desire to have a sense of the world in terms of motives and a simple tendency to choose positive intentions rather than hostile ones are strongly linked to the essence of our changing mind. This is the basis on which adult morality is built.

In summary, it is safe to say that human inclinations are not exclusively egotistical: friendliness and altruism have evolutionarily been valued in friends, and even children sometimes try to help!

Does Human Nature Exist

There are many cultural and personal differences between people, but have people anything intrinsically in common?, no human nature exists. Under his opinion, the mind is a "blank slate" without rules when it comes to conception, so data is introduced, and guidelines for their care are only created by sensorial experiences.

Even if he was incorrect, we could have a human nature that seems complicated.

"Although we're prone to violence, we're also inclined to compassion, to teamwork, to self-control." (Steven Pinker, professor of psychology at Harvard) So the word "human nature" is ambiguous, because the question is whether such a thing exists or not. Does the sentence lead to what it seems to be? Was humanity a misnomer or a true idea?

Is the nature of man an animal?

Biology sees people as just another animal species — one with the greatest intellect and the highest order. As animals, we aspire to satisfy our innate needs for food, drink, shelter, and sex, as well as a fundamental need for physical comfort and pain avoidance. In The Selfish Gene, the biologist Richard Dawkins points out that our human make-up must have had a selfish nature to be healthy enough to live over the centuries.

On the other hand, although we have done it to the detriment of others because of the achievement of our predecessors in fulfilling their bodily needs, it is difficult to see how the whole picture can be this kind of human essence. Biologists find it difficult to describe altruism and empathy to some people after natural disasters, which requires an aspect of self-sacrifice.

Is human nature basically good?
A famous Chinese philosopher, Mencius, thought that goodness arises from innate human tenders toward benevolence and wealth, for example. He argued that an individual's bad behavior, rather than his or her constitution, is due to an unhealthy environment. Contemporary secular

13

humanism holds a similar view. For example, it is thought that people turn to crime because of poorness or because they conform to their delinquent subculture. Humanism demonstrates a belief in the inherent goodness of human nature by its focus on the importance and effectiveness of human beings.

Nevertheless, in view of people's inhumane and humane behavior, it is difficult to maintain this view.

"The human nature is potentially violent and destructive, potentially organized, and positive." Is the nature of man inherently bad? (Margaret Mead, cultural anthropologist) Both religions have the belief that the true nature of people is false. Nevertheless, the definition approaches what I view as an extreme version of' original sin' in the Christian Orthodox doctrine. The Catholic Church and most major Protestant denominations believe that all people are born in a sinful condition as a result of Adam's sin.

14

This disorder has in many respects been defined, from a propensity to sin but without collective culpability, to something as extreme as total depravity or universal blame by the collective error of all humans. In my view, this theory has contributed to an overwhelming personal sense of guilt and self-denial.

Another theory is that our normal state is to be conscious that we are a separate, self-contained entity, with our own mind and body. The effect is a general self-orientation tendency. Part of our composition is, therefore, a natural concern for one's own needs. This can be a positive thing, like with social skills self-development or self-reflection of inner feelings. The problem is that if we are not on our guard, it can mean self-indulgence and a selfish attitude.

So we are not born inherently bad nor basically good in line with this view, but our human nature consists of both positive and negative patterns.

Another exception to the purely natural desire of human nature arises from religious reasoning on clearly human faculties. The theory goes back a long way to ancient Greeks. In the works of Plato and Aristotle, the human soul has a divided essence. Another aspect is human and moral, in particular. Another segment is home to impulses or interests like animals.

In a similar vein, , we human beings, in comparison to animals, are able to think with autonomy and moral discernment, and thus to be human is free and to think and to choose rationally. "To try to figure things out is human nature. So, when we are in a state of affairs, we usually try to reason through it. What is more human than the capacity to look down on ourselves, so to speak, to our sentiments and thoughts, and apply ethical principles? If we want to, it allows us to understand more deeply meaningful and valuable things. There is no animal that has this self-aware, reflective existence. Therefore, we humans do not need to imitate instinctive and conditioned responses blindly. Alternatively, we have the freedom to follow some of our natural inclinations in this or that direction.

They should cultivate potential human qualities such as empathy, compassion, and kindness for others. But how does that happen?

One solution is to recognize, in our lives, what comes from outside but can be present in us - the Divine Origin of all that is good.

Understanding the Flea Life Cycle to Help Plan Control Strategies

A basic understanding of the flea life cycle is useful when preparing a flea control strategy and when more control measures may be needed. The cycle of flea life is the basic process of insect life, which includes four main phases: adult female fleas lay flower eggs on the cat. These fall away from the animal into the environment, where they have flea larvae- the highest concentrations of flea eggs are in areas where pets spend the most time, such as litters and recreation areas.

Flea eggs is a thin, white, worm-like phase (about 5 mm) feeding on dog's or cat's debris like' dirt' flea. Flea dust or feces are a nutritious meal for larvae because they are high in protein and not digested entirely by the adult flea. They are generally not seen as they leave deep in a layer of carpets or pet bedding. After maturing, they turn a cocoon around to form a pupal stage.

Flea Larva pupa is identical to a moth's cocoon phase. The cocoon is very difficult to kill with insecticides and is vacuum resistant because the pupae bind tightly to tap fibers and animal bedding. If a dog or cat is not available to feed (e.g., when households go on holiday), the pupal stage can remain sleeping for a long time up to 150 days.

Flea Pupa This phase can also create a reservoir of floats that can infect animal animals long after an active flea control product has begun to be used. Pupaes need the right stimuli such as vibration and carbon dioxide from the object that passes by to hatch out of the cocoon. When this is happening, they spring and leap on the animal quickly. If the family is on holiday and the house is huge empty numbers of starving, unrefined fleas will float simultaneously and stick to animals and even humans.

18

Adult fleas leap into an animal as immature fleas that feed very fast and are usually attached to the animal within one minute. We are ready to eat for the first 24 to 48 hours. This prolonged feeding is required to provide protein and energy needs for the preparation and laying of eggs. She is ready to lay eggs once a woman flea has been on her animal for 36-48 hours. For up to 100 days, she will place about 20 eggs per day on the coat of pets that is about 2000 for every person!

So what are some important tips on flea control that we can learn from a flea life cycle investigation?

If you wait until you see many pulleys, you ask for trouble before using an effective float control product. Each female has laid 20 eggs each day, so you already have an infested world when you start treatment. Start an effective flea control item Before you plan to see fleas before the weather gets very hot. Don't be surprised if you see flues for weeks (up to 8 weeks) on your animals after you begin using an efficient flea control item-the pupal stage may be up to 100 days without taking any blood meals-so there might be a wide pool of pre-emergent fluff waiting to jump on your dog. Both fleas in the world also have to go through their life cycle and become immature adult flutes that infest your pet before they are killed.

The pupal stage is very resistant to chemicals, and therefore, it will be much more important to focus on the use of an active ON ANIMAL flea control product than trying to control the life stages in the field.

If your home or yard is riddled with fleas, do not limit your treated pet's movement. When you think there is a horrible flea problem in your pet's dormitory, please keep letting your pet go in. A properly treated dog becomes a mobile flea killer. If your pet is not allowed in an infested area, hungry fleas will try an alternate blood supply-either you, your family, or your mates! Yet we know that flea eggs are collecting where your pet spends most of its time-be sure to focus on cleaning and vacuuming these areas.

Ensure your use of an active flea control item is optimized. Make sure you dose your pet correctly and follow all the guidelines on the product label.

If you have some of these ideas from your experience of the flea life cycle, you must be well-positioned to handle these poor little pests. Good luck in the war over your flea!

Who Wants "The Good Life?"

People regularly talk about the good life as though it's the best thing since sliced bread. In principle, I would concur totally. The main issue is that the majority of us do not understand what it means and notwithstanding for the individuals who understand, it's still a battle to manifest.

You might get a wide range of ideas of what the characteristics of the simple life are; nonetheless, I speculate they would all point to a specific something - Happiness. At the point when it's everything said and done, we all need to be happy.

Imagine that - living a happy life. It sounds extraordinary - sounds simple as well, isn't that right?

Why at that point is it so hard to achieve? I have taken a gander at this from such a significant number of points and still have no unmistakable response to this puzzling question. Of course, there are true principles, and a right value framework that plays big comes in an individual's happiness BUT, what are the roadblocks?

In my experience, there are numerous roadblocks; in pretty much every case, paying little mind to what our barriers are, we frequently make them. Indeed, even in situations where some other person or thing is responsible for the roadblock, our response to these things is the genuine reasons we succeed or fail.

So at that point, what is The Good Life and how would you achieve it?

Life is simple

The first thing that I have come to realize is that life is SIMPLE! Seriously - people toss the term around freely - be that as it may, it has demonstrated to be true again and again. Every one of the complications we face in life is either made directly by us or by our response to our circumstances.

Pause for a moment - close your eyes and think about it. Consider it long enough, and I believe you will arrive at a similar conclusion.

When I state life is simple, here is the thing that I am genuinely getting at...

Life is simple when these 3 undeniable values drive it:

1. **The choice-the minute that you realize that everything is precipitated by choice**, possibilities become interminable. The word cant cease to exist in your world, and you consistently observe the light in each situation. Unquestionably, you may have down days; be that as it may, generally, you are the quintessential optimist.

2. **Purpose-a life of purpose is a life worth living**. When you understand that you have something unique - that we as a whole do - to offer the world, you begin to understand your purpose. Besides, when to make choices that lead you to live right to your use, you mostly lead a purpose-driven life. Nothing is more fulfilling than knowing that what you do has value and that you are here, which is as it should be.

3. **Others-life is simple when we serve others.** When we make choices that lead us to fulfill our real purpose, and that purpose makes and distributes value to others, we genuinely are living a full life, a simple life - a good life. You can't desert an incredible inheritance in this world if nobody other that you were in an ideal situation for you having been in it.

At the point when these 3 values are grounded in and directed by right principles - when you abide by natural laws - life is GOOD!

What stops us?

EVERYTHING! At the point when our choices and actions are not driven by our core values - mainly the 3 above - and grounded in the right principle, life instantly winds up complicated.

I challenge you to think of any situation where you settled on choices that were out of line with your core values and did not abide by natural laws, and I guarantee that you will find some complication.

Life will never be simple as long as we are misaligned. Negativity spreads most feverishly when we are lopsided. It breeds frustration, dread, outrage, and desirously among numerous other pessimistic emotions.

Since these are on the whole emotions, we can exhibit as well as control. It is precise to state that the main thing that prevents us from living a good life is us. YOU are the one stopping YOU.

If you find it hard to believe this simple truth, the good life will, without a doubt continue to escape you.

We are altogether brought into the world with everything we have to live a plenteous life - we are in truth all intended to do as such. It doesn't make a difference where you are from or how you were raised - YOU can pick your very own way. Life is the thing that you make it and not the other route around. Regardless of who or what you are blaming for your station in life, if you continue, I guarantee you that nothing will change to support you. You are simply the one robbing of the fortunes in your life. The minute you realize and believe this simple truth, you will experience an immediate, significant, and positive shift in your life.

Again, I am sure you will have awful days - we as a whole do; notwithstanding, your belief that you can change any situation in your life to mirror your true desires will dependably be sufficient to turn things around. It never fails!

Simple isn't in every case, easy.

A wise man once said, "simply isn't in every case, easy." In my experience, this is right on target - no question.

For instance, we, as a whole, realize that we ought to eat healthily, but then the more significant part of us don't do as such. A few of us are more outrageous than others, yet I am sure that we've all succumbed to our taste buds, notwithstanding when we realized we should state know.

In other instances, numerous people smoke since it feels better while they are doing it. Of course, they all realize that smoking is terrible for them, but then they still do it even though they know it takes a long time off their life span.

Both of these are simple truths that we as a whole know; nonetheless, such a significant number of us find it so difficult to do the simple thing - it merely isn't that easy.

The way that simple is in every case easy, however, can't be a reason give up on living the good life. We deserve to seek after it consistently. Besides, if you are not living "The Good Life," it means that you are unbalanced with your core values and true principles.

There is nothing good about living if you are not happy and you are of no value to anybody. Regardless of whether that kind of living feels suitable for some time - it will keep going for some time. It will, in the end, erode your inheritance and nobody will recall why you were here.

CHAPTER TWO

How To Live an Abundant Life

To different people, abundance means different things. It's really a nice holiday for some, and it's a sports car or a large house for others. And that's my first argument. Abundance is whatever you can achieve. And that can be a material possession, a friendship, a friendly attitude, health, joy, or anything you want.

Why have some people got the big house, the happy relationship, enough money in the bank? This is because, in their lives, they have prepared themselves to experience these things.

If someone sent you a check for $3 million tomorrow, will you probably accept it? But are you going to feel confident about it? Or would you believe you don't deserve it at some level? There are a lot of people out there who would feel more insecure because they don't think they've done enough to get so much for' nothing.'

Nevertheless, the World is vast. There is no shortage, and the idea that we must work hard or even work to be worthy to obtain is unfounded. Beliefs about wealth can take several different forms, including "I don't deserve to grow money not on trees," to "money doesn't make you happy."

Through economic, love, passion, wellness, friendship, family, etc., you attract into your life is all a reflection of your state of mind. It's not a product of the school you attended or the college you attended. In today's World, there are many examples of people with very limited education but who are some of the richest on the planet. There are examples of people who have cured by the power of the mind from incurable diseases. All these are living witnesses of the power of the mind and the way our lives are made.

Abundance is related to the way we see our lives right now. So basically, it's down to seeing the glass half full or half empty.

Are you a person who focuses instead on what you don't have? The rule of the Universe says you will get more of what you focus on. When you dwell on your mortgage, talk of hating your old car, focus on everything that's wrong in your relationship, and then you get more of this because it is so easy and strong that the Universe answers your thoughts.

Create a dream of what you want to attract in your mind. Keep it as vivid and dynamic as possible. Also, cut out magazine pictures. Write down how you want your life to live on a piece of paper. Don't include material possessions only. Write down how you'd like to feel like your normal day. You're employed, you're raising a family? Have you a lot of friends, live in the city or in the countryside? How much cash have you in the bank? And when you wake up, how do you feel? Build the vision — Essential-Write down what you want exactly as if you have it already. Remember, the Universe literally takes your thoughts. So, if you write,' I will live in a big country house,' it will always be a vision for you and stay in the future. In other words, in your present life, it will never materialize.

Be happy once you have developed your new dream of how you want to live your life. Be grateful for all you already have. Be grateful for the food you can consume, for your friends and family, for the TV, and even for the rusty old car on your drive, or your safety. Even if you don't feel good, your body keeps you alive. And thank you so much for that!

Thanksgiving is one of the main powers behind abundance. If you want to attract more to your life, be deeply grateful to have it already in your life. And by first class mail, the World will put on its skates and send more to you.

What you have in your life at the moment is a product of your past life. This can be a divisive assertion most people don't like listening to. It is far more appealing to the ego that other people are responsible for what we have, conditions beyond our control.

How to Live Your Purpose

It is my fundamental belief that every one of us has a big definite meaning in our lives in this universe. Everyone has a unique destiny to contribute with their unique mixture of skills and interests to this world. I have no doubt that most people are working hard today and staying busy with everyday activities. The issue I have found is that many people live their lives without any real purpose that brings motivation and importance to their lives. We are interested in the daily mechanical processes of life and rather than purpose-driven creatures. It might be the most important thing you will ever do in your life to find and form your main purpose, because your intention is to build all your accomplishments, and it provides the boundless source of inspiration that drives you to achieve all your goals and to allow you to live life in full.

What is a major purpose?

Your main purpose is like a path you follow on your long life journey. Your intent is something you are very passionate about by its very nature. Yeah, the juices only flow in order to pursue it. This guides you through your acts and motivates you to do what you do, in spite of the hardship and the pain you may have to face to do this. Think back to the history of all the historical figures. What was the meaning of their life? You will note that throughout history, the great people have so strongly believed in their mission that some have died in the search. That's how big your target must be. You must be willing to trade the rest of your lives happily in the pursuit of your important purpose.

Why are some people experiencing a mid-life crisis?

Even if we do not describe our meaning clearly early in adult life, at some stage between the ages of 35 and 50, it hits most of the us-the notorious midlife crisis. This "crisis" almost always comes from an inner voice that tells us that our lives are missing. This feeling is the necessity to find and pursue our definite purpose in life. It is our unconscious mind that says,

"Hey, you are already at this halfway point. Why don't you stop wasting time and start to do what you should be!" Why wait for your subconscious alarm clock? Right now, start working on it.

There is an important distinction to make between goals and your real purpose in life. Your most definite purpose is NOT The goals. Your purpose in life is not your goals, but rather determines all of your lifetime goals for yourself. In your life, your purpose is like a queen ant who creates all the soldier ants in the colony. Those soldier ants are your goals, and without them, there can be no ants colony, and likewise, your life will have no meaning without a queen (his purpose) to carry these goals forth. So they're going to go hand in hand.

 How to get what you want— faster than you ever thought possible, it says that your goals in life must be precise and measurable according to the same standards as your goals. That's something I tend to disagree with. Your main goal should be a lifelong journey of dedication without a clear pause. The explanation for this is that if you set your definite target with a realistic objective such as the main definite goal was to invent the light bulb, then what can you do with your life after your purpose is finished? Anthony Robbins predicts that many adult males will die within a few years of retirement, not because of old age or poor health, but simply because they have nothing to live for anymore. The purpose does not follow the same standards as setting goals. There is no concrete endpoint for your intent. The measures used in measuring your performance are dictated by how people regard you at the end of your life. How many lives are you going to save, touch, and encourage in your life? How's history going to judge you? When you are gone, what things or people are you going to leave behind? The legacy you leave behind is the measure of success in fulfilling your primary purpose in life.

How to define and explain your purpose in life in six steps In the discovery of your purpose in life, there are two sections. The first part is your general-purpose, which is basically how at the end of your life, you want to be remembered. The second part of the exploration of your target is how you plan to achieve your general objective with your unique gifts, skills, and abilities.

Phase 1-Take your work daily routine social retreat. Finding your life purpose is perhaps the only one most significant response you will find for yourself, and it is fair that you need to devote 100 percent of your mental and spiritual energies to that effort to find your meaning. With all the turmoil in our everyday lives, it is not even realistic to try to find the meaning of your lives when juggling the other obligations. Take a few days and go on your own private break. Go to a quiet and peaceful place where you can really see your main objective. Step 2--Identify your core competencies. Make a list of eight things you really do well. These can include your own abilities, expertise, and skills. At this point, don't worry about your purpose. Only mention the best of your skills. My core skills include writing, coaching, and teaching.

Step 3--Identify Your Happiness. Make a list of four things you love and want to do. These are things that you would happily do without compensation because they provide you with endless joy and happiness. The passions list would probably be a copy of your list of core competences because you usually do what you also enjoy. Contrast your core skills with your passions. Now you have a list of four good things and the things you want to do.

Phase 4--Identify your ancestry. Your legacy is how you want to be remembered after you have left this world. What are your contributions to society? Brainstorm a legacy, write eight suggestions, then use a tournament drawing system to give your list priority to the most significant legacy. This can be done simply by combining the eight ideas and choosing which of the two is most important, and then repeating it "tournament," until you have a winner. The winner is your ultimate goal in life.

Step 5--Link your passions to your target. Note that it is not sufficient to make a general-purpose relevant. You must also determine what tool you are going to use for this reason. Our goal could be to help others, but our approaches could be very different. Simply evaluate your list of interests and core competencies to learn how you can use them in your life to achieve your goal.

Step 6--Build a Statement of Purpose. Your personal statement is a concise statement as to why you are here in this world. It consists of two parts: a general objective and a method. Keep your statement of purpose as concise as possible and limited to just two sentences. Your first statement is what you want to do with your life–the legacy in Step 3. The second sentence is how you intend to achieve this–your method. My personal statement has always been to help as many people as I can realize their personal dreams. I achieve this by writing, coaching, and teaching others how to maximize their potential.

Dedicate Every day to Your Purpose Once you have defined and explained what your purpose is, you have to dedicate yourself to this path. This can be easily achieved by doing something every day that pushes you toward your target. While those acts are small, if each day you do at least one thing which gets you closer to your goal, then by the end of the year that is 365 small steps. You will have taken 10,950 moves towards your main purpose by the end of 30 years. No matter how small those steps are, they will add up as time advances–so start today! When going to sleep at the end of each day, ask yourself if you have given yourself everything that you had to give that day.

Create a mindset never give up the path to your destination is never an easy one. Inevitably, you will face challenges, some minor, some very rising. Regardless of the challenges you face, it is crucial that you cultivate the courage to do whatever it takes to achieve your ultimate goals in life. Adversity will test your resolve, and it is up to you to lift the sword and battle every obstacle.

Random Thoughts On Life And The Human Universe

Sometimes you have a new thought, idea, or eureka moment, but it's not bodybuilding enough to turn into a good essay. So there's a potpourri of thought about life and the human World (even if not all of that) that's too interesting not to note, but not enough food to eat.

Life Defined: Presumably, there are as many different definitions of "what is life?" as scientists, life scientists, naturalists, and philosophers, etc. Many focus on or around concepts such as development, reproduction, stimulus-response, metabolism, second law violations (entropy), and related ilk. None were entirely sufficient; otherwise, we would have the description of a text. My interpretation of "what's life?" is slightly different. Life is a kind of complex organic structure that has nature that is not completely predictable by classical (or even quantum) physics. And, in other words, the' structure'

41

will do as it wishes in the most tightly regulated and consistent set of laboratory conditions!

Life: There is no such thing as "living matter" or "dead matter," speaking of life. All matter is deceased matter as all matter consists of protons (gluons and quarks), electrons, neutrons (more gluons and quarks), neutrinos, photons, etc. All matter is "dead matter." Few if anyone would argue that the' living matter' is an electron, proton, neutron, etc. Yet atoms are not alive, therefore molecules, even complex molecules. Everyone is alive or' living material.' No matter. The "alive" is the framework, the configuration of different parts and parts of the matter, in very particular structures, so that chaos, at least temporarily, is thwarted-and that's the key point. Entropy succeeds when the organizational structure disintegrates, i.e., life dies.

Death: Death is not a matter of fear. You're dying, but not death because once you've been gone, you don't exist, and you need to live, to live everything, something, even death. So you're not dead, only to death, but not to death.

Afterlife: it's clear the fundamentals of the things that make you, you-personality, intelligence, imagination, feelings, intellect, memories, etc.-are changed, ranging from pain, sleeplessness, food chemistry, alcohol, drug, and other chemicals inhaled, ingested or otherwise absorbed into your body. The nature of what makes you are therefore based on physical fact and, therefore, on physics (and not only on gravity). So unless science and physical processes are supported by the home(s) of the afterlife and there is a physical mechanism that can transfer your physical soul from your body to a dwelling that supports physical afterlife, otherwise you forget about life after death.

Afterlife. You don't want actually to die, but you don't want to really want to have an everlasting future. I say, after the first million years, you would be bored with billions and trillions of years to come, which is just the beginning! Sounds like hell to me a little more! Your future will happen within the Earth, somewhere, but what happens in your afterlife, when the World is finally dead or explodes in a Big Brunch (in

43

comparison to the Big Bang). Regardless, it's your future curtains. It's also clear that your body doesn't go afterlife when it dies. If you're going to an afterlife, you will make the journey through your spirit, your consciousness, and the meaning of what makes you. Nonetheless, how about a one-day-old child or for a 110-year-old who has extreme dementia or for someone from moderate age who was an ex-boxeror ex-gridiron-player with such a pumped head and brain that he is just a fraction over a vegetative state now. The same could happen to someone who has been starving for a long time for oxygen, such as an almost drowning victim. What about your future with a nine or five career, a boss with a lousy band, a large amount of email and an unproductive and useless workload, loads of bills, taxes, and a golf course, as well as the lawyers and the horrible family. Add a supreme deity to that mix who cracks the whip at all hours. Speak of the pre-life now. Wasn't it quiet, peaceful, and tax-free? What if your post-death was like your pre-life, wouldn't be "Heavenly," and now it's just someone else's question, as an additional bonus.

Meaning, intent, and nature: The frequently asked question is: "What is my life purpose? Why am I here?" People want some kind of significance and meaning to their lives and often try to offer religion. That's pure faint-heartedness. The World offers no sense to you. The universe does not allocate any meaning to you. It doesn't matter to the World why you're here. The World is not a superpower because the universe can't give a goddamn in the sense that a rock can not give you and your search a goddamn thing. You don't enter the heavens or fall from the high Ten Commandments style and say why you are here and what your intent and significance is. If your answer to why you're here is intent or intention, it is because your own purpose and meaning have been given, but perhaps through loving others, including family, educators, spouses, etc.

* *Plants*: people call them weeds. Mother Nature names plants to them. The so-called "weeds" are also part of the natural scheme of things. Stupid people!

Evolution: If species A is responsible for Species B, it's extremely unlikely that Species B will appear anatomically and

45

mentally in just ten million years, dramatically different from that of Species A. Evolution takes place, but gently, softly, step by step. In ten million years, a species of cockroach won't turn into an ant or spider or fly. After ten million years, a stegosaurus won't become a parrot. The human species also needs more reasons in contrast to a chimpanzee or a common ancestor of chimpanzees. We look and act in the time available just a little too far away.

Human Species: Although it is true that some others can sometimes walk upright on two legs for brief periods, only a bipedal human may climb up or down a step and balance a tray in one hand while thinking about something else, like sex and not falling down. Only a bipedal human can maintain equilibrium in comparison to our primate cousins while dancing or playing games that involve quick and rapid transformation. But a bipedal position is almost like a hand on its side. It's very easy to fall, boom.

Human Species: Given the very common yet self-promotional conception, the least rational species on this planet are human beings. Any other animal behaving irrationally, whether through a genetic defect or illness or dementia equivalent, is a dead animal. I still have to witness any animal that has any form, shape, or form, which is not rational for its own survival or for the survival of its genes, community, or kind. I certainly can't say the same about the species of humans.

Human Species: Human beings and cycles go hand in hand with a hat. Although the majority of the systems are artificial and, therefore, somewhat telephonic, cycles are important for people and human society. The day-night cycle is of paramount importance and a natural cycle. People have a lot of money in the seven day week period, an artificial city, and to a smaller degree in the month (also a phony cycle that is so loosely based on the lunar cycle). The year is a natural cycle (in seasonal terms) and probably the most important year next to the day and week cycles. Decades and decades are rather meaningless and in any case, artificial. The millennia become significant only when the calendar changes from 1999 to 2000 (though the current millennia, in reality, started in 2001), and 1000 year periods are nevertheless outside human life. And that should be quite so-apart from some ancient societies with seemingly important cycles, which pre-existing (and concluded well after the societies had been extinct), such as the Mayan long count (recognize the famous date of the doomsday of 21 December 2012). Many cultures calculate on-going cycles of devastation in such long periods that they do not have an immediate effect on their propagating societies. When communities have phases of significance without immediate value, you have an anomaly and have to wonder where this particular cyclical definition has been given.

Human Language: Modern people are one species, several races, but one. Nevertheless, our single species is in use and extinct in thousands of languages. This is a phenomenon. Phenomenon. Other species, each one of which is indifferent races such as cats, dogs, and horses, have a special vocal language (complemented by a body / facial' speech,' as in the case of humans). A Chinese cat can chat, which he understands with a French cat, an Egyptian cat, or an Australian cat. Why people needed or developed an enormous number of spoken languages alone is a bit of a mystery. On the other hand, the' language' of the body/facial is quite basic and therefore singular.

Human body: Perhaps you think of yourself as a special species. The words "me, me and I" are all special. But you know perfectly well that you are actually a colony of thousands of organisms (cells) working in total harmony more often than not. Yet you are housing billions and trillions of bacteria as things turn out. Nine out of ten microbes that make up you aren't really part of you, like the surviving and thriving bacteria in your mouth. So, are you an organism, an organism colony, or an organism-environment? I'm shocked to know that 90% of me isn't me! So perhaps our true purpose in life is to represent the larger crowds as hosts. The needs of the many[microbes] are greater than[human] needs.

Diet: That we have everyone's read and heard how we consume far more salt than essential and too much salt could exacerbate heart and blood pressure and correlated nasty conditions.

*** Diet*:* The feedback mechanism to restore the right balance is never stated in all these health warnings about salt. It is close to how many bars can provide customers with free salted chips or salted peanuts. It isn't out of bartender's sheer goodness. When you get a lot of salt, surprise, thirsty. And so the bar sells the' free' peanuts and chips by selling more drinks to quench your thirst and eat all the' free' salty stuff. In other words, if you excessively indulge in the salt, you will have more liquids because you are extra thirsty, and the excess fluids will take unnecessary salt (salt urine) until absorbed through the kidneys, and the balance is restored. And, if we drink a lot more salt than is required, we probably drink a lot more fluids.

Archeology vs. Mythology: There is a large number, as this well-known Stegosaurus at Angkor Wat, of old rock gravings or petroglyphs and so on, of what seemed to be dinosaurs. Creationists use these images as evidence to show that dinosaurs and human beings coexist, actually, categorically. Skeptics have the notion of a field day, but those photos still exist and continue to be explained. My right! My honor!

Now, mythologically in the World of all things, there are depictions of hundreds or hundreds of imaginary beasties (carvings, paintings, rock art, statues, etc.), often of animal-human hybrids such as the centaur; hybrids like dragons and griffins of animal animal and other plain beasts such as the thunderbird, or those that are plain bizarre, like the bulls with the flute, etc. Such mythological beasts are often shown in everyday settings cheek-by-jowl with real animals as usual regular. Besides deer, foxes, goats, cows, gangs, and cats and dogs, you'll be as normal-just like that; Stegosaurus has truly modern creatures that have been carved in relief in Angkor Wat.

No surprise, IMHO, is that by chance some of these mythological or imagined beasties, creations or constructs of the human mind would just turn out to look like actual, albeit long extinct, forms of life. And if we see a rock formation that looks like a stegosaur, it is just a coincidence.

Archaeology: The Australian Aboriginal: With respect to the Australian Aborigine, why no aboriginal culture was ever presented to me by the Great Mystery? In other words, Aboriginal people had the knowledge and the ability to build things (with a cost of 50 000 years). But there is no

51

equivalence of American Indian mounds or pueblos. No pyramids or temples, no likeness to a Stonehenge or Newgrange, no likeness to a statue of Easter Island or a large wall or an army of terracotta, certainly not something similar to ancient Greek /Roman buildings. Yes, the Aborigines never even had anything as important as pottery. Why? Why? It seems to me to be a huge phenomenon.

Archeology: The Wheel: when you look at the most important and fundamental inventions, only a few people really stand out. Fire taming is one. Cutting devices like flakes of stone is another. Writing is third. Writing is third. The thought of nothing or zero was a real breakthrough. And there's the drum, of course. There are, however, a few irregularities in the rim. For example, in ancient America, the wheel was both known but not used. Translated, you find children's toys with wheels in the archeological record. What you don't consider is the definition extrapolated to the realm of adults. The wheel was used in people, be they Incas, Aztecs, Amerindians, etc., even when wheeled toys prevail. Now the basic reason is that they did not have beasts of burden such as crates or horses to pull wagons, etc. However, that does not explain the fact that the wheelbarrow or small wheeled wagons/carts/ platforms or shopping carts or the even primitive rickshaw can be pulled by a single person is missing other practical application for adults. Not all wheeled must be the size of a chariot, a covered vehicle, a stagecoach. Even a potter's wheel doesn't work, and so on. The idea of rounding or rolling (as in logs) is evident to the most fundamental societies, and yet the super-civilization, at least at that time, of ancient Egyptians, was not used for the first half of their very long reign. There seemed to be no wheel-eureka moment for Australian Aborigines either.

Archaeology: the Orion belt: consisting of the three bright stars Alnitak, Alnilam, and Mintaka, the stars in a straight line are more or less evenly divided, thus being visualized as a belt. For some mysterious reason, the trio of stars that make up the Orion Belt shows or reflects many archaeological sites. The trio of these huge ancient Egyptian pyramids on the plateau of Giza is the most famous. The second is the main pyramid complex in Teotihuacán in Mexico. The third is a Hopi Mesas set in Arizona. Sure, Orion's Belt is quite prominent in the night sky, the stars trio, but then too many other star patterns.

Which makes our ancient ancestors special? Much of this is achieved by' late astronaut ' theories. Somehow this trio of stars must be unique, such as ET house turf. Sadly, everything that doesn't seem possible. There are also bright stars: Alnilam (Epsilon Orionis), Mintaka (Delta Orionis), and Alnitak (Zeta Orionis) but also very, very far. That alone means they're very un-Sun-like. Alnitak sits at a distance of 736 light-years and 100,000 times the brightness of our Sun; Alnilam is 1340 light-years away and 375,000 times brighter than our Sun; and the Mistake lands 915 light-years away as the crow flies, and the brightness of the Sun rises to 900,000. Mintaka is also a network of double stars. The trio of stars making up Orion's Belt does not seem likely to be candidates for aliens, who would be deemed "old astronauts." I am very skeptical that SETI scientists will consider these stars as likely candidates for radio telescopes.

Virtual (Virtual Reality) Universe: In a virtual world scenario, I (and many others) have indicated that we existed as a software program or subroutine in a larger software program on a computer. The undefined conclusion is that the Supreme

Programmer is of flesh and blood (terrestrial or alien). But why do you say that? Why not say that the Supreme Programmer was/is an innovative artificial intelligence. Silicium and steel (artificial) intelligence is a rational evolutionary counterpart to flesh and blood (natural) intelligence and is not just likely to evolve much quicker (Moore's law) than human evolution ever did but to have a wide range of durability.

The Basic Kabbalistic Understanding of Human Nature and the Nature of Our World

We can see if we get a better understanding of the nature of life and the complexity of our universe, with all its laws and facets. Therefore, we can also resolve the problems of our lives first and then push toward a much brighter future.

The study of various substances shows that each matter and object's primary purpose is to maintain its existence.

Nevertheless, in each material, this concentration is expressed differently. Strong objects have a fixed and defined structure, which makes it difficult to penetrate the "boundaries," while other types defend themselves through motion and transition. We must, therefore, ask ourselves what makes a substance act and distinguish from other materials in a certain way? Which governs the behavior of every form of matter?

Substances ' action is somewhat like a computer screen. The picture on the monitor may impress us, but a computer expert treats the same picture as a mixture of colors and pixels. The technician is only interested in the various parameters that generate the image. Computers realize that the software picture is just the superficial presence of a specific combination of these powers. We know that elements have to be changed to give a clearer, brighter, and more precise image.

Each entity and every structure represents its special, intrinsic combination of forces in nature, including human beings and human society. In order to cope with any specific problem, one must first understand the behavior of matter at various levels.

And in order to do that, we must go deeper into the underlying power that matters.

The will of existence The intrinsic strength of each subject and object is usually called the "will to exist." It designs the form and the quality and behavior of substance. There are infinite ways and variations of the will to live that is at the root of all the material in the universe. A higher degree of a substance represents a greater desire to live, and the various desires in every degree (silent, vegetative, animate, and the talking (human) of substance form the different processes.

The Desire to survive is based on two principles: 1. Keeping its current form, ensuring it remains; and 2. Including something he thinks to himself is important to his life. The ability to add something to itself varies between the different degrees of matter.

The first degree of Desire: let's still look a little more closely at this. The smallest Desire to survive is still at the point. This is because the needs of the still are limited and need not add something external to themselves to survive. His only desire is to preserve his present form, structure, and qualities. It also opposes something new. Because its only wish is not to change, it is still called "still." There is a stronger desire to exist on a vegetative level. It's fundamentally different from the quiet urge because the vegetative changes, and they still don't change.

The second stage of Desire: the vegetative does not "settle" like the still to maintain its life, but undergoes other processes. The vegetative attitude to the world is therefore involved. For example, plants move to the sun and send their roots to humidity sources. The vegetation depends upon its existence— the wind, the rain, temperature, humidity, and drought. The vegetative receives its environmental specifications, decomposes them, and creates from them all that it requires. Then it secretes and grows what is harmful to it. The vegetative form is, therefore, far more dependent than the silent on its environment.

The vegetation has its own cycle of life– Plant Live and die. However species one of the same are rising, thriving, and dropping by the same rules. In other words, all plants of a certain formwork in the same way, and there is no individuality of certain elements in the genus.

Third desire level: animate The more a will for a form exists, the more reliant it is on the environment and its response to it. The relation becomes more apparent in the animated class, where the Desire to live is greater than in the vegetative. Many species live in groups, in packs. They are highly mobile and constantly have to travel in search of food and appropriate living conditions. Animals eat other animals or plants and use them for their sustenance as a source of energy.

The animate degree reveals the same degree of personality development, which causes individual sensations and emotions and gives each animal a unique character. Every animal senses the environment individually, gets closer to the beneficial, and moves away from the harmful. The animal life cycle is also human. Every individual lives and dies in his own time, as opposed to plants whose life cycle is determined by yearly season.

The fourth level of Desire: human The degree of human will is the greatest degree of the will to live. Man is the only fully dependent being, and the only man feels the past and the present and the future.

The climate is influenced by humans and the environment. Therefore we humans are constantly changing, and not just because in our present condition we are happy or unhappy but because our knowledge of others makes us want something that others have.

Therefore, we want more than others or not, thus improving our situation compared to others, and increasing our sense of self-gratification.

Throughout humans, that is why the urge to live is called "ego," the Desire to enjoy or the Desire to obtain happiness and enjoyment, as Kabbalists term it "the will to receive." Rabbi Yehuda Ashlag, revered as Baal HaSulam, says that: "the

Desire to receive, was from the beginning to the end, the whole essence of life.

Humans are not only a slightly more advanced living thing; they differ profoundly from the animated. At birth, a person is a helpless person. Yet we rise above all other creations as we evolve. A newborn calf and a mature bull are largely differentiated by their sizes, not their intelligence. Nevertheless, a human baby is practically weak and completely helpless. But it slowly grows and develops over many years. Therefore, the growth of a young animal is very different from that of a human child. Our sages put it as follows: "A calf of the day is called an ox," it means that, once a calf is born, it is considered an ox, because as it grows, it has little substantial qualities.

Unlike all other animals, humans need to evolve for many years. It doesn't want anything when a baby is born. But as it grows, its ability to obtain increases and expands enormously. When a new need arises, the human being feels compelled to meet new needs. In order to meet new desires successfully, the brain evolves as we start to consider ways to satisfy the new need. The cognitive and mental growth of the brain is, therefore, a result of the rise in our ability to enjoy.

We can see how this idea works by studying how our children are brought up. We build challenging games to help you develop, and your desire to succeed in the game makes you think of new ways of coping that will make your progress easier. From time to time, we make the game harder to help them develop and keep progressing. Therefore, when you believe something is lacking, you can never grow. Only when we want something do we start stimulating our intellects and pondering how we can fulfill our desires.

The fact that a man is both intellectually and emotionally composed improves our willingness to receive, as mind and heart complement each other and enhance our perception of things that can cause pleasure. Therefore, our willpower is not time or place constrained. For example, we can not feel events that occurred a thousand years ago, but we can (and do) understand events of the past so that we do not feel them.

Therefore, we should get ourselves to the point where we really can understand them through our intellect.

The alternative is also possible: we can evaluate the situation positively or negatively with our intellect and link it to our perception of the object when we perceive something and want to explore it. Therefore, mind and heart expand our perception of time and place until we are endless. A person living in a certain time or place would, therefore, want to behave like someone he or she had heard of, even if there were a great distance, either in time or distance, from the object of such admiration. That is why people want to be like great historical figures often.

When we are fulfilled with our will to obtain, we perceive it as enjoyment. We feel empty, depressed, and even begin to suffer when we can't satisfy our desires. Because of this, our happiness depends on whether our needs are fulfilled or not. Every act we can do, from the simplest to the most complex, is done only to enhance satisfaction or reduce pain. These are just two sides of the same coin. In his essay, "The Peace," Baal

HaSulam says, "Natural scientists know it's not possible to make even the slightest move without encouragement, which means that one has no gain. For example, if you move one' s hand toward the table, it's because you think one's hand will obtain more gratification by putting one's hand on the table. In reality, our ability to enjoy is the inner engine that drives us forward and triggers the processes that take place in human society. We are constantly evolving our desires and designing our present and future.

The Cycle of Life is the Secret to Balance

Surely the best thing is that it all changes. This is the nature of our universe of vibration. Life consists of cycles, and these cycles are the catalyst for continuous transformation and spiritual growth.

The world in which we have been born is the pinnacle of what the human race created as a group since the human species evolved to the point of cognition and awareness.

Our earliest ancestors acknowledged and accepted three facets of our being and, as part of their culture and rituals, thanked the origin of all life. The life process is one of constant transition and shows the belief that all things pass in cycles like tides.

Existence in the physical world has brought us to the point where the main focus in existence is on the mind and the body. We are at a critical juncture in our growth, which needs us to return to the power of the spirit of our creation. The power and balancing perspective of our spirit is necessary not only to balance ourselves but also to balance the common part of human experience.

In the mind, body and spirit triad that is our essential nature, we need balance. We will put the calming power of our mind back into our cycle of decision-making moment by moment. We have to do this individually and collectively.

But this is the contract. We can only do this collectively by personally first "being it."

65

Don't talk about it as something to do. Think of this as "something being." First, you must "be compassionate" to do merciful things. You must first "heart" to do loving things. You must first "be noble" in order to do noble things. You must first "be the truth" to do true things.

Were you "the facts" of who you are? Or are you "the reality" of the idea of who you claim to be? Who you really are is a product of God's spirit. This is the ultimate truth of you and of every existing human being. We are all God's holy kids, and as such, we all belong to God. Not only some of us but for us all.

We are all one. Just most of the time, but always. We are all working gigantically with Him. In the physical realm, we perceive all that God knows as ideas in the absolute sense.

If you experience the belief that you are separated from God and a fear of God in life, well, that's all right. You have free will to experience and believe anything you want.

Just one thing I want to ask you. "Does that represent you?" Does this make you think that you are a separate person from everyone else, so it's all right to kill your mates if they disagree with you or have something you want? (Like olive oil).

Will it help you to believe that you are removed from this supporting earth, and you are therefore entitled to contaminate and kill the very environment that keeps the filters to cleanse the air we breathe and provide the pure water of life?

Does it benefit you to think that you are a different being to yourself and are separate from the source you come from and, by believing in this isolation, you have denied yourself the power you have as part of this omnipresent and caring source?

This belief in distance from any and all things and people and God, at this particular moment of human existence, is the most common belief amongst most people on this planet. Here's the good deal, though. It's just a belief. That doesn't make it a reality.

Before this separation system of belief became the dominant system of belief in this world, there was the prevailing belief that we all belonged to the sacred and benevolent essence of the origin of all things. This was a millennium ago when most of the world's communities were matriarchal, and the idea of religion was not really developed.

Such early societies were not warlike, and they provided for all society members. We considered every person a worthy part of the whole and valued the world as a life-giver.

The human cycle is no different from any other life cycle. When tides come and go, the cycle of life also takes us to a point where the faith in separation must give way to the faith in unity and allow mankind to once again step into the healing ways of nature and unity.

CHAPTER THREE

Life Cycle Cost Analysis

One of the most important considerations for energy-saving or green building stakeholders is to know if and when the investment will be worthwhile. In order to attract investors, guarantees must be provided that their investment is profitable. Investors, stakeholders, and project managers use various instruments to measure fiscal feasibility, and the Life Cycle Cost Analysis (LCCA) is one of the most effective ways of determining total costs.

LCCA is a form of assessment that takes account of the financial dimensions of construction project acquisition, ownership, and execution. Project managers can also help to identify alternative possibilities and focus on achieving project performance objectives. The Power Life Cycle Cost Analysis (ELCCA) approach can be used when comparing two or more design options. ELCCA is a computer model that quantifies various design alternatives accurately.

Federal Requirement

LCCA uses systematic evaluations and comparisons of possible building design alternatives to identify the best choices for total cost-effectiveness, including ownership, operation, and maintenance of a specific building. This implements a set of methodologies for life cycle costs and procedures in compliance with the Code of Federal Regulations (CFR) and forms part of the Federal Energy Management and Planning System. LCCA regulations follow energy conservation policy standards, including the NECPA and Executive Order 13423, also known as the Federal Law on Environmental Strengthening, Energy, and Transportation Management.

Purpose of LCCA

Various costs can be found in green-building projects that will ultimately decide the total cost of ownership of the project. These include initial procurement, purchasing and construction

costs, operation, maintenance, and repair costs, costs of
renovation, disposal, energy costs, financing costs or payment
of interest charges, and other non-monetary costs incurred by a
project.

In short, LCCA is used as a method for evaluating the overall
cost of each design alternative to determine the option that
offers the lowest total cost of ownership without compromising
quality and usability. LCCA is used for each design alternative.
When performed in earlier project phases, particularly in the
design process, project managers are able to choose which
alternative results in the lowest life cycle expense.

The Benefits of LCCA

LCCA are not only applicable to green building projects, but
also to decision-making regarding investments inland. It is very
useful to define what building alternatives can deliver the most
economical long-term model. This makes LCCA a better tool
than other approaches that concentrate on first costs or short-
term costs associated with transactions alone for the detection
of total costs of ownership.

To show the benefits of using LCCA, we will decide whether it is more cost-effective in the long term with high-performance HVAC or glazing. A crucial part of the process is to take account of both short-term and long-term ROI costs. High initial costs can often be believed to outweigh long-term benefits. This is not always valid, and the LCCA approach will prove that. It is also worth noting that LCCA can be extended from start-up to attitude to various levels of complexity in the project life cycle.

ELCCA and Green Building

ELCCA may be a powerful research and decision-making method for choosing the most cost-effective device choices when evaluating energy use in refrigeration, heating, boiling, lighting, and other operations. The ELCCA modeling study describes and proposes the safest and most sustainable development alternatives for green buildings in terms of energy quality, comfort, productivity, and occupant safety.

ELCCA is implemented as a non-static system and is continuously improved and updated as new alternatives are discovered and adopted. The final design can be a mixture of a number of decisions based on the ELCCA method of classification and choice. Such correlations and conclusions are properly documented in the final ELCCA report with the related effects.

A Natural Life Cycle of Human Being

Composting process A transition from life to death and back takes place again in the soft, warm bosom of a diminishing compost heap. Life is leaving yesterday's crops, but in their death, these leaves and stalks transfer their energy to future generations. The wheel of life is spinning here in a dank and moldy heap.

Compost is much more than fertilizer or a soil wound healing agent. It's a sign of a lifetime. Before man first walked on this planet and before the first dinosaur raised his head over a primeval marsh, nature made itself a compost. Leaves that fall to the forest floor and gradually rot are composted. The dead grass of the meadow sewn by the winter freezing is exacerbated by the moisture of the earth below. Birds, insects, and animals contribute to this extensive and continuous system of natural soil reconstruction.

Compost Heap The compost heap in your garden is an amplified version of the process of death and rebirth that takes place in nature almost everywhere. In the process of running the organic garden waste from various types of leaves, grass clippings, weeds, twigs are always collecting, and since time immemorial, gardeners have collected this material in piles, finally spreading it again into the field as thick, dark humus.

Composting is practiced in many parts of the world today as it was hundreds or even thousands of years ago. Farmers and householders in Asia, Africa, and Europe in less developed areas have no source of commercial fertilizer and thus make rough piles of compost of cattle manure, refuse, waste, straw, and weeds. Such piles compost into humus and are then used for the kitchen garden and farm fields as a soil conditioner. Compost of this kind is not too rich in plant nutrients, but it is a manageable type of humus that maintains the tilthy and overall condition of soil used for generations.

Garden waste products can be turned into a brown, fragrant, crumbly, or partially decomposed organic substrate called compost in many ways.

The aim in all composting is to organize organic waste so that soil bacteria and fungi can thrive and increase when they break down them. The bacteria are the raw material converters and must be in a workable environment. You need humidity, ventilation, and food.

Basic process Make the compost with a mixture of green and dry materials. Grass clippings, green weeds, berries, pea, and other tasty materials contain bacteria's excellent bacterial sugar and protein. We are easily decomposed. Savings, dry leaves, twigs, and prunings contain very little nitrogen and gradually

75

decompose alone when composted. What you want is a combination of green and dry.

Gardeners also found that the best way to build a compost pile is to place between layers of waste material, a layer of mixed fertilizer, manure, and garden soil.

You start the pile by spreading a 6 to 8-inch deep organic waste layer. Spread the mixture of manure, garden soil, and fertilizer over this layer. Manure and a commercial fertilizer should be used to provide bacteria with the requisite mineral nutrients. The higher the fertilizer, the better is the compost. A decent average of 2 cups of ammonium sulfate or blood feed per square foot in each sheet using more for the dry waste, less green stuff.

Fall the fertilizer surface down to bring chemicals into the ground; do not clean with strong watering.

If you apply a cup of ground Silestone, crushed oyster coating or dolomite lime to each layer, you will find a less acidic material in places where the soil is on the acid side. Add another vegetable layer, spread over it the chemical soil manure layer, and wet it down. Continue the layering cycle until the pile is 4 to 5 feet high.

Hold the stack as wet as a sponge. Water may be required every 4 to 5 days in a hot, warm climate. The thickness of the wood content can affect the degradation rate. When dry leaves are poured into the pile, the decomposition is much slower than the shredding of the leaves.

Under normal circumstances, the pile should be rotated 2 to 3 weeks after starting, then every five weeks. It should be able to be used in three months.

Fast high heat process The time for compost can be shortened to a few weeks if all the waste is shredded before the pile is built. Since more substrate is exposed to growing bacteria, the smaller pieces degrade more rapidly. Shredding also allows a fluffier mixture that facilitates more effective absorption of air and water. If you don't rent or buy a shredder, shred all large leaves with a spinning mower.

When the weather is warm, when the pile is installed, you will see thermal waves in 24 to 30 hours. Turn the stack to blend the material and water thoroughly. It will warm up again and be hot enough in a few days to transform on. Whenever you turn it, move external materials to the center, where heat and humidity encourage decomposition.

The destruction of most of the weeds is a clear advantage of this fast, high-heat composting method.

Once it's cooled, the compost is ready for use, dark and rich in color, crumbly and with the scent of the good ground.

It is worth splitting into three batteries or compartments in your composting area. The first one is for routine collection of organic waste vegetable garbage chopped paper, collection, coffee plots, eggshell, kitchen vegetable pelts, mild pruning, wood ashes, and green or dried weeds. The next compartment is for the working compost, which is not supplemented, but the principle is regular turning. The third compartment is for the finished or almost completed item

The Basics in Healthy Longevity

For decades, the human race has found ways not only to extend its life span but also to make older years healthier and more successful. In the first Biblical book of Genesis, we read about people who are literally centuries old, who have children when they're well over the age of 100, and who have hard work (Noah was 600 when he and his three sons built the ark), when they were several centuries old. When someone lives to 100, they receive special letters from the queen, president or prime minister of their country and congratulate them on their long life. In early Biblical times, they were considered pure young people. The obvious questions are, "What is the reason those people in Genesis can be living so long and are able to duplicate it today?" Many people have claimed that the word years really should be months, which would mean that Noah if taken as an excuse, was only 50. Nevertheless, this theory has some issues as we, for example, "As Enoch had 65 years, he was father of Methuselah," which implies that when we use it as the theory of the year every month, Enoch was just under 5 and a half years old, when he was a father, an impossible biological thing, of course. And we accept the word year again to mean exactly that, 365 days of time. This then takes us back to the question, "Why did they live so long?" Several hypotheses were raised to explain longevity, including the following: 1. Toxin-free environment reduced the rate of airborne diseases and emissions 2. Diets were much easier without cooked, fried, or modified chemically 3. 3. 3. The genetic pool was much purer at the time and contained a variety of diseases and disorders today.

5. The lifestyle of the people was much slower and had no pressure whatsoever today.

5. The people were much fitter because they had to do it all by hand and walked about.

While each point is true, it still lets us ask: How can we use this knowledge to help us live longer today? We recognize that aging begins at the cell level and that the cells are less able to reproduce healthy cells as they mature. We must find a way to reverse this trend and regain the cells ' ability to reproduce healthy cells.

Looking back on the above list, we can see that each of the five points would create less pressure on the cells in the body, which in turn would allow them to grow healthy cells longer. But what we have to do is to try to replicate these conditions as closely as possible so that our body cells can continue to reproduce healthy cells longer.

When we started at the first point, the environment was much better, we need to find ways of cleaning up the air we breathe, and to do this we have a wide variety of air filters available for use in our homes and workplaces. It certainly would help the cells to be safer. Of course, it goes without saying that we would not be a cigarette or smoker around us while cleaning up the air we breathe. That's known as staying away from the earth if you really want to live longer. It refers to the smoking of anything.

Furthermore, we should look at the things that we consume and remove refined, fried, and chemically modified meat from our diets. We should instead eat fresher, raw, organic fruits, and vegetables. They should also ensure that high-quality vitamins and minerals are adequately balanced so that cells have all the nutrients required to grow healthy cells as well as to carry out their job. Another very recent discernment is RESVERATROL, a substance found in red grape skin that has been found to provide many benefits for your health, including extending your lifespan, protecting your heart from infections, preventing and battling cancer, and increasing the metabolic rate that allows us weight loss. This should definitely be part of the supplementary curriculum for all.

Another element of supplements is the preference for natural products rather than medications. Most physicians don't treat causes, treat symptoms, and prescribe another drug for each new symptom you create. Please realize that each drug has its own side effects/symptoms and is liver toxic. So if you really want to get your body clean, you have to get rid of the toxins that have build up in it over the years and substitute them with natural supplements that really help the body's healing efforts and enhance its safe lifespan. There are several ways to obtain toxins from cells, such as the use of some plants, ion foot spas, and colonic/colonic washing, the removal of toxins is an essential part of living longer.

Thirdly, the integrity of the genetic pool could be a concern because the genetic defects we have inherited can not be prevented. Through working to improve our own wellbeing, however, we will actually pass on a stronger genetic code to our children than we did. Therefore, if we teach our children to live healthy lives, they will transfer an even greater genetic code to their children than they have from us. As this trend continues generation after generation, people will live longer and healthier lives.

Fourthly, with respect to lifestyle, we also make a number of different choices about how much work we do and how quickly we spend our leisure. Stress on the job may be inevitable, so give your body, mind, and spirit a break by providing recreational activities that can de-stress your cells. Part of this stress reduction technique is to ensure that you sleep well during the night, with your head and neck well supported. You should sleep at least 6 to 8 hours each night. In the morning, you will feel refreshed, stress-free, and ready to enter the new day. Shift workers who often have difficulties getting enough sleep live ten years less than non-shift workers on average. If we work during the day and relax at night, our body clocks work best.

Another thing to bear in mind is "electrosmog," the electromagnetic fields which always surround us from the appliances, computers, mobile phones, lights, and every electrical gadget we use. As several studies have shown, the high frequencies they produce have a direct and negative impact on cell safety. For example, people who use cell phone forms for an hour or more a day are 75 percent more likely than those who do not use or seldom use cell phones to develop brain cancer. Scientists at the Israel's University of Haifa have also studied nighttime light and cancer satellite measurements in 164 countries. The highest rates of prostate cancer were in the brightest countries, more than twice those in the dimmest nations. In another study, Harvard researchers found that people with the smallest night melatonin levels are 60 percent more likely to develop breast cancer (postmenopausal women). When light suppresses the brain's melatonin production, the more likely a woman's chance of developing breast cancer becomes. It highlights again the need for six to eight hours of sleep every night.

To enhance the body's capacity to withstand the harmful effects of the electromagnetic frequencies, we must reinforce our cells, just as we get from the magnetic field of the planet, by safe low-frequency electromagnetic frequencies. Surfing the sea is a very healthy exercise to help strengthen our cells against harmful frequencies. For those of us who can not touch the sea, we use pulsating electromagnetic field(pemf) equipment that provides a complete range of electro-magnetic frequencies in our body cells that every cell type must be safe.

Fifth and last, is the need to exercise our bodies. Our bodies are made to move, and it's a sure way to lower cell health and cut our lives not to keep our bodies going every day. We will perform aerobics for at least 20 minutes at least three days a week if possible weekly. It helps our bodies to maintain good cell health through increased circulation, which leads to providing nutrients to every cell that we discussed in part 2. The use of pemf increases the cell's ability to absorb at least 50% nutrients, which obviously can only produce healthier, more robust cells.

A Primer for Longevity- Aging Gracefully

The human body is a development marvel. Our cells are built with a genetic blueprint for building and maintaining a fully grown adult human. If your field of work is kept clean and all nutrients provided, our cells continue to perform their job perfectly. And much longer than you could imagine. Current thinking suggests that the human body was genetically engineered for 120 years. So why do many of us get on the scrap pile and sputter in the 1960s and 1970s to a humiliating conclusion? The explanation for this is more because of poor maintenance or the way we live our life than because of our genetic condition or a mystical biological clock.

In other words, people would live longer if they took better care of themselves. A lot longer. A lot longer. It is never too early to start to plan for a healthy future. If you have something of 30, 40, or 50 years, the information in this section can make the difference between graceful and safe aging or pain prematurely.

"In the natural universal order of things, with our aging, we get older, two things of biologically critic significance are occurring to accelerate aging. The rate of increase in the number of cells destroying free radical reactions is significantly increasing. It sounds like a fair age until you consider a recent Surgeon General report, which concludes that 80% of Americans do not die of old age. These were destroyed by degenerative diseases. Diseases such as cancer, cardiovascular disease, diabetes, and arteriosclerosis. There are no people who develop degenerative diseases like coldness. Over the years, we give them poor living and unsuitable eating habits.

The aging or senescence of our cells is mainly regulated by two factors. The inheritance (our genetic composition) and the impact of internal and external elements resulting from the way we live our lives (the food we eat, the air quality we are breathing, the stress we have in our bodies) depend on the number of times the cells are scheduled to replicate them (genetic potentials) and how much time they are between generations. The time frame is not in stone. The longevity and replication levels of cells are greatly affected by lifestyle factors such as stress and the nature of our food.

Most people are fatalistic about how long they live and about their quality of life prospects. The risk of this action is that it allows them to relinquish their own responsibilities. For example, "If I do nothing, I'm going to die anyway?" Indeed, there is ample evidence that we can affect our degenerative disease capacity, enhance our longevity and increase our length and quality of lives-regardless of the quality of the health of our parents or the length of their lives.

Smoking, excess alcohol intake, rancid and oxidized fats, food additives, nutritional nutrients deficient, overfeeding, pressure, and pollution all speed up the aging process.

Polyunsaturated fat from vegetable oil is one of the main culprits and can become very quickly rancid. This fat quickly absorbs oxygen molecules and produces hydroperoxide lipids. Such molecules break in our bodies and release very strong free radicals that cause a chain reaction of destruction. The overall mortality rate caused by these fats is even more prevalent than cardiovascular or vascular disease. The most popular sources of these fats are corn, safflower and sunflower margarine, shortening, and salad oils.

Monounsaturated fats, on the other hand, slow down the aging process. These are slow to oxidize, limit free radical reactions, and decrease the LDL cholesterol level. Avocados, Macadamia nut oil, Olive oil, olives, flaxseed oil, almonds, and hazelnuts are the best foods sources. Researchers in cholesterol, Ancel Keys, outlined the argument for monounsaturated fats when he revealed that Mediterraneans with the lowest death rates use olive oil as their main source of fat. They are less likely to die of anything prematurely.

Another problem with oil is how it is used. The cooking of beef, poultry, and even fish, when browned, produces compounds known as heterocyclic amines (HCAs). Through animal studies, HCA has been shown to cause colon, breast, pancreas, and bladder cancer. It activates free radicals and destroys the genetic material (DNA) of the cells. High-temperature cooking, including frying, grilling, grilling, and grilling, is mostly HCA-producing. Roasting and baking produce little HCA and stewing, boiling, and wildlife virtually do not produce HCA.

Low removal and toxic accumulation cause a huge amount of premature aging. At the Rockefeller Institute for Medical Research, Dr. Alexis Carrell took small bits of heart tissue from a chicken embryo to create one of the most impressive medical experiments in history. He tried to show that the living cell could survive for very long, even forever, under suitable conditions. The heart tissue was plunged into a solution of nutrients from which it received its meat. Interestingly, waste material has been secreted into the same solution. Every day the formula was modified, waste and fresh nutrients were added. This chicken heart tissue worked in this way for 29 years. One day, a worker forgot to change the metabolized polluted water. It died. Self-intoxication declared this great masterpiece of scientific experimentation. "The cell is eternal, just it's the fluid in which it floats, which degenerates," Carrell said. "To resuming this fluid at intervals gives the cell something to eat, and to the degree, we know that the pulsation of life may go on forever." Poor diet· Lack of physical activity· Emotional or psychological stress· Medicines· Lack of adequate water To enhance elimination eat plenty of high-water and fiber content foods, drink plenty of water, make sure that your diet includes plenty of minerals (especially magnesium)· Lack of food and drink plenty of fiber The colon is good health food, with super greens, extra vitamins, flaxseed tea, flaxseeds, bran, whey, brewers yeast, yogurt, and leafy greens.

Low digestion and absorption extract the vital nutrients they need from the aged bodies. The human body is an entity that retains itself but can only repair itself if it receives the requisite raw materials. Digestive enzymes, HCl, and pancreatic enzymes can be used for good digestion and absorption, but it is best to chew your food carefully for proper digestion.

One of the powerful things we can do to delay aging and boost health is to eat a low-calorie food diet. There are more people over the age of 100 on the island of Okinawa than in any other country. We eat 17 to 40% fewer calories than other Japanese people and 30 to 40% less cardiovascular diseases, strokes, obesity, diabetes, and brain diseases related to age. That's just the reverse of how Americans eat (low nutrients, high calories). Excess calories are the enemy of youth because it takes more oxygen to turn them into fuel and unleash free radicals (a natural metabolism by-product). The freer the radicals in our bodies, the more harm the body can do. Restricting calories by consuming less but thicker nutrients decrease free radical production. Experiments have shown that underfeeding animals have higher levels of antioxidant enzymes and have 1/3 of the immune systems of such food animals than normal animals. The response is to eat whole foods that naturally contain low calories and high nutrient content.

The following are the keys to a longevity diet:· Eat a total of five to nine portions of fruit and vegetable a day (serving 1/2 cups of cooking or chops, 1 cup of raw leafy vegetables or 1 piece of fruit)· Eat both raw and lightly cooked (fresh is the highest in antioxidants, but cooking gently helps to absorb nutrients· Eat brightly colored vegetables and fruits.

Grapes-contain 20 skin and seed antioxidants. The brighter the hair, the more antioxidants it contains. Orange and violet grapes are better than white grapes.

Grapes-3 to 5 times as much antioxidant content as new grapes· Onions-full of antioxidants. Onions prevent cancer, increase cholesterol in HDL. Red and yellow onions are the best quercetin food in the world that inactivates anti-inflammatory, anti-bacterial, anti-Hungary, and anti-viral agents.

93

Spinach-high in lutein and beta-carotene decreases cancer risk, heart disease, high blood pressure, strokes, cataracts, degeneration of the macular tissues. Spinach decreases by 25 percent the chance of macular degeneration. It is also high in folic acid, a safe brain, and artery· Tomatoes — the best and only trustworthy lycopene source that maintains mental and physical workings among the elderly. High lycopene blood levels reduce the risk of pancreatic and cervical cancer and other digestive tract cancers. Cooking tomatoes and canning will not kill lycopene.

Eating food rich in antioxidants is smart, but it makes even more sense to limit the production of free radicals. An individual can do a lot to limit free radical development in their bodies. Exercise puts the system with more stable oxygen. Poorly oxygenated tissue is more likely to cause free radical damage than healthy oxygen. Air chlorine, plant contaminants, and smog are all skin harmful. You may not be able to do much with smog, but you may drink clean water and eat organically grown food. Pressure encourages the development of free radicals, so learning to manage stress is very important. Keep your intestines healthy. The colon creates more free radicals than anywhere else. Keep it clean and run smoothly. Repopulate the colon, a natural enemy of pathogenic bacteria, with bifidobacteria. Get enough sleep. Get enough sleep. Melatonin is released during sleep, a potent antioxidant. Not only does sleep regenerate tissue, but it is also important to remove free radicals from the body. Drink lots of water. Drink plenty of water. It helps to remove the harmful effects of an excited oxygen form called singlet oxygen (a free radical). If we drink enough, this free radical is absorbed by water and is harmless. It will hurt the tissues if we don't drink enough water.

Jean Carper says at Stop Aging Now,' Aging-the adverse changes that happen in the older years is, in fact, a major, progressive disease of deficiency. As we get older, our bodies are becoming fewer and fewer able to extract nutrients from our food as our dignified structures degrade with age. Zinc deficiency can cause or exacerbate arthritis, depression, degeneration of the macular, and poor immune functions. 40% of 51 and older people don't eat enough. Appetite can cause 30 to 50 mg of zinc a day.

B vitamins are important to keep our minds sharp as we age. Niacin has shown that it prevents and even reverses senility symptoms. 100 mg works a day, as does avoidance. People with low B-12 levels and folic acid have a poor cognitive function, as well. Dementia and depression were shown to improve with-12 treatments and the treatment of folic acid.

A Harvard study of 87,000 nurses found that the major heart disease events (the number one cause of female death) were decreased by 41 percent for women who took vitamin E from 100 to 250 IU a day for two years or longer. These also reported a 29% lower risk of stroke and a 13% lower overall mortality rate than females without vitamin E supplements.

Antioxidants block radical damage free of charge. Within their molecular structure, they have an extra electron to give up without becoming unbalanced. We produce fewer antioxidant enzymes as we age, so if we want to remain healthier, we want our antioxidant intake in food and supplements to be increased. Vitamin C, E, beta-carotene are the most common antioxidants.

Zinc, selenium, folic acid, B-6, manganese, and magnesium are provided. It is a good idea to use a variety because they function in various parts of the body. For example, vitamin C neutralizes free radicals, and pycnogenol works more closely in the connective tissue. Polyphenols and bioflavonoids have powerful antioxidant properties in many herbs, spices, fruits, and vegetables. Eat lots of fresh fruits, berries, whole grains, raw nuts, and seeds. Limit metal. Unless you're a kid, a teenager, or a child-bearing woman, you probably don't need any extra iron. Excess iron is much more likely to make you sick and old than keeping you young and healthy, especially in past middle ages. Iron turbocharges free radicals and increases their aggression and destruction. Iron transforms harmless cholesterol into the form that affects the heart and arteries. If you have high cholesterol, it is particularly dangerous to have too much iron. In a Finnish study in 1992, men with high levels of iron are twice as likely to have heart attacks than men with low levels of iron. Stay away from extra iron–cut down on animal products and iron-fortified cereals to reduce free radical activity.

CHAPTER FOUR

Human Life Expectancy

Were you aware that significant progress in biotechnology, genetics, and medical sciences is now rising human life expectancy ever more rapidly?

What that means is that those of us who are 50 or older and in good health and live in a developed country can now expect 30 to 35 years of working life after retirement. What are you going to do with this third stage of your life?

The good news is that the internet revolution has given older people many more opportunities and greater flexibility to earn more money and to keep up their sense of purpose and meaning in their lives.

The "retirement" in this era of the longevity revolution is not the end. It is a new beginning, and what you are making from that new start will be in all your pockets.

How much time can you live?

If you're really Fifty yrs of age in a developed country, the average life expectancy for 2011 was around 81 years, when we are between 85 and 70 years old. Now that is based on the actual age-specific death rates in 2011 in the population, and it is undoubtedly a very conservative estimate considering the levels of positive change that are already happening in biotechnology and medical science.

The Future of "Retirement" Life

Let's look at how life can become a true reality for the elderly. The most important change, if we were to retire at 60-65 and lived for 100 years on average, is that 30-35 years of potentially active and productive life are ahead of us.

The great news is that "retirement" is not the end of this new age; it's really a new beginning, and what you're doing about the new start is totally in your hands. That's an exciting prospect, I think, don't you?

now I'm sure, and most of us all want to spend more time together with your family and friends, visit places we dream of seeing, renovate our homes or move to a smaller, more manageable building, just relax and reduce our stress levels and spend more time on hobbies and interests.

But many of us want more if we're 30-35 years happy and successful! Those of us who've already led a busy life, and we're diligent and concerned about a good career, will not just quit. In reality, it could be a very bad thing to do in terms of our potential life expectancy.

It is true that we need a strong sense of purpose in order to preserve our passion for life, our sense of identity, and meaning. Throughout our working lives, these conditions are fulfilled by our jobs, our families, and our relationship with our partner. Now the career is over, our kids are most likely grown up, and our relationship with our wife is also changed, as we are spending more time together than we have in the past. We will work hard, adapt, accept, appreciate, and redefine all partners.

Internet Revolution has also changed anything.

So, what could we do to protect and preserve our sense of purpose and our passion for life and keep income flowing? The good news is that everything has changed in the internet revolution. So we still now have many more choices in life, and it is easier more than ever to create a new company by using the power of the internet. We can, therefore, keep working, and raising extra money in our later years-which we might need because we are living longer, safer, more productive lives. So we can work at home or beach, anywhere in the world, and for the hours that suit our lifestyle, and we can do everything in the best way by pursuing our passion for life.

I think, with 30-35 years of active working life ahead of us, many of us will want to go back to universities and prepare for a second career. Can our "retirement" take one or more years off from work to retrain us for our new careers? Going back to college can now be as simple as turning on and connecting to the internet.

Major progress in biotechnology, genetics, and medical sciences is now rising ever more rapidly with human life expectancy. And we 50 years of age and older can now look forward to 30 to 35 years of active life after retirement in good health and living in a developed country.

This new third life phase provides us with the opportunity to enjoy a completely different retirement from any previous generation, with new challenges and exciting opportunities. The good news is that the internet revolution will provide older people with many more ways of earning money and maintaining their sense of purpose and value in their lives. "retirement" is not the end in this time of the Longevity Revolution, it really is a new beginning, and you will make this new beginning completely in your hands.

Retirees Face Serious Longevity Risk

The danger of longevity: the danger of survival... that is, a threat of running out of money before you breathe. This is the number one concern of the majority of pensioners... and for a good reason. A retreat can take 30 years or more, and it is a lifetime that can reach very expensive medical emergencies or that a sudden collapse in the economy will rob you of your financial resources. If you add to the risks of your fixed savings ' diminished buying power triggered by inflation, higher real

103

estate taxes, lower interest rates, and incapacity to operate, Longevity Risk is easy to understand by a majority of pensioners. We can do little about unemployment and taxes, other than wisely using our votes to pick fair, loving politicians. Health can be controlled somehow by eating correctly, exercising, and not using excessive smoking and drinking in our bodies. They can not do much to be removed or regulate the economic cycles and interest rates from the labor market. Ultimately, the only thing we can monitor for sure is how much risk we take to our pension funds.

If your pension money is in a risky place, such as the stock market, and a crash happens, then you are possibly going to suffer a significant loss without any way and time to do it. In reality, if you lose your retirement money because you have played and lost on the market, there will be no second chance... you will depend on the government, your family, or an advocacy group. Not an appealing thought and probably the main reason most retirees say their number one fear is to live longer than their income. Too many retirees did not, sadly, take action to reduce their investment losses by going to safe places. Why is this? Why?

Next, you are bombarded with ads, advice, and commitments to keep your money on the market. You are advised that, with shares, securities, mutual funds, complex portfolios, and other risky investments, you are going to be more successful in "long term" than if your cash is being held in safe places such as bank CDs, government bonds and fixed annuities. You have slick graphs and maps showing how much more you can do with your money at risk. The whole brokerage industry relies on you to bring your money on the market and to make sure they work really hard. You can not read a newspaper personal advice column, watch the news or read any of the thousands of magazines or newsletters dedicated to finance, without advising you that your retirement money is better off by making it safer on Wall Street. You never remember the collapse of the market between 2000 and 2003, or the early 1970s, nor do you remember that Wall Street is currently suffering losses due to its profligate activities. The broker is constantly calling how the time to buy at cash prices is now.

What about your losses already? You are scared to accept that you will not make a reasonable return because you put your money at risk. In reality, you are told that you'll realize your biggest fear of outliving your money if you keep your money super safe. The truth is, you are much more likely to survive your money by taking risks, which you can not afford than to keep it super safe and earn a security interest rate. Note, the risks and rewards of traveling companions are always: if you have a chance to make a big return, you take the risk of failure. On the other hand, the gain will be good and certain but not above-market if you take zero loss risk. What do you like, then: the chance of great growth, but also the risk of major losses OR absolute security and a small but certain return? As Will Rogers once said, "I'm more interested in my cash than in my money's return." I believe Mr. Rogers was right about the standard retirement.

The current economic situation is not that reassuring: unemployment is rising, the dollar is low and dropping, the oil spills nearly $100 barrels, the housing market is totally deteriorating, subprime lending issues are spilling over into cars and credit cards, inflation is growing, and deflation is being widely spoken about. The Federal Reserve, the nation's currency protector, is clearly terrified by the drastic move that has taken place during the last few weeks to push short-term interest rates into the basement rapidly. Many analysts, including me, are pessimistic about preventing a nosedive of the economy: depression is what I see. Yet you currently have the majority of retirement assets in mutual funds[check your401(k)], stock and bond portfolios, and other risky investments. Have you forgotten the events of the bubble dot.com? Have you been worrying about what you would do if the economy fell sharply? Should you know that if you lose too much of your retirement money, you will not have a second chance? What can you do? What can you do?

One choice is to look for a stable lifetime income that you can not maintain. You see, longevity insurance is available: the insurance companies that are some of the largest, best, and oldest financial institutions in the world are prepared to guarantee you a lifetime income that you can not lose by depositing your pension money in them. You must bear the

107

market risk, valuation declines in shares, real estate crashes, and other unforeseeable changes that can wipe out your retirement money. You still have taxes, inflation, health issues, and non-investment risks, but you can't survive your capital. How can such promises be made by insurance companies? The way you protect your house, your car, your safety, your career, your company, and other valuables: the rule of the greatest number and the hazard distribution. When you live too long and lose money in ensuring a lifetime income, someone else in your community does not live as long as you planned. The average numbers are. Therefore, time-consuming and the insurance company can manage the risk and make a profit. On the other hand, you were shielded against your most frightening retirement risk: the survival of your money.

How do you know more? Tell the financial advisor to speak to you about a lifetime guarantee that an insurance company has secured. By the way, once you start speaking about "variable annuities," tell him or her you want something safe: discuss a fixed annuity, without any adverse risk and one that allows you to begin, stop or store your lifetime guaranteed income. To get a guaranteed lifetime income, you do not have to give up control of your assets because insurance companies have started to offer new services, which specifically address longevity risks to retirees in recent years. You can change your mind with these new plans if your circumstances change. Insist on stability and insist that there are no business risks. If you do not want to look into the option but leave your pension funds open to the market, make sure that you have a clear answer to the question: "What will you do if the worst case is real?"

Will Your Retirement Savings Survive Longevity and Long-Term Care?

You should have resources allocated to your future retirement when you reach the age of 40 years. It takes some effort to plan a successful future retirement. You should use the 401(k) option of your employer. They should make efforts to save money in an IRA because your company does not provide a401(k),403(b), or a fixed pension program. You can start a

SEP account if you are a self-employed person. Planning, however, does not end with saving money.

Which happens when your health improves because of a prolonged illness, an injury, or the consequences of aging? As you get older, these health risks significantly increase. Will your pension plan last long?

For many Generation X and Baby Boomers, retirement planning has become a top priority with long-term care. Most individuals from 40 to 70 years of age have directly discussed the consequences of long-term health care to their families or others.

The concern is that too many people are forgetting to cover pension funds against rising long-term care costs. You, your family, your economy, and your lifestyle will be impacted by the financial costs and the costs of aging.

70% of your lifespan will need a certain form of extended care. Looking for your parents is very difficult. It is not a good plan to rely on your children as caregivers. We have their own jobs, families, and commitments or will have them. It is not that they do not love you, but it's difficult to have a son or daughter or a solicitor. It can also affect your health and employment.

Spouses are also not a good care choice. When you mature, they do. We will also have to deal with their own health and age issues.

Paid treatment drains your wealth and impacts your income and lifestyle adversely. The costs of long-term care and support continue to rise. Even a growing nest egg can be affected.

the current national average care cost at home is $4,195 per month. The cost of a living facility dependent on support starts at $4,000 a month before you begin adding facilities. Skilled home care costs $8,365 a month–more than $100,000 annually. Long-term care expenses increase over time.

Most people mistakenly believe that Medicare will pay in the future, pay for long-term care needs. Health insurance,

Medicaid, and supplements only pay a limited quantity for qualified professionals-and only if you change. Such insurance options do not cover the cost of custodial facilities that assist in everyday activities. Many people, however, require custodial services when they grow old.

While the longest-term treatment arises when we are older, people of all ages require extensive care. Early-onset dementia, even in your 30s, will occur, including Alzheimer's, the most popular form of dementia. Multiple sclerosis, Parkinson's, and even strokes occur at younger ages. Today, your good health gives you the chance to plan ahead.

Medicaid will pay for long-term care, but you need to be poor or end up being sick. It is something you want to stop for most men.

Ultimately, the investments and families are affected by the financial costs and pressures of aging. Affordable long-term care coverage covers your wealth and eases the pressure on your family otherwise.

Although some claim that long-term care coverage is expensive, it is actually very affordable for most people, especially if you prepare before you retire.

If you're well enough, these plans will match many people's budgets easily. Too many people are looking for assistance from a financial advisor or general insurance broker with little information. Sometimes they make recommendations which are too large or sometimes too small. Therefore, many of these practitioners work only with one or two insurance companies because they don't have a good understanding of how policies are used when they say that their advice is out of line with what you really need.

In addition, 45 states are offering long-term care alliance programs that provide direct dollar-for-dollar asset protection.

In most countries, there are several types of policies. This includes traditional plans, partner plans for the additional protection of assets, single premium' hybrid' plans that also

113

offer a death benefit, and short-term plans with broader age and health qualifications.

The key is partnering with a specialist in long-term care insurance who deals with major insurance companies. I still ask several extensive questions in order to draw up an appropriate proposal on the specific concerns and budget of the client.

The prices for long-term care facilities vary from place to place. Many arguments begin with care at home, and many people avoid a nursing home because they get the right attention at home or in a sponsored living room. Those rates are far lower than professional care in a health care facility.

Long-Term Care Insurance will pay coverage at home, adult care centers, help facilities, memory programs, and conventional skilled nursing homes. You and your family determine, with most plans, how you use the benefits.

Will Long Period Care Insurance work? Definitely. Absolutely. In 2018, major insurance companies paid US families over

$10.3 trillion in premiums. Otherwise, these families would have had to drain their own assets to pay for treatment, become caregivers, or both.

As policies are tailor-made, you can decide what is important for you. The important thing is to prepare before retirement. Long-term treatment is not sexy. It doesn't shine like a new car or a new diamond. Perhaps you won't show your agenda at a party. However, it will give you and your family peace of mind.

Working with a specialist in long-term care would help you to obtain accurate information. Start your research in your 40s and 50s if you have the cheapest options.

Long-term care coverage is simple, affordable, and has a steady level of income and asset security.

Managing the Employee Life Cycle

Does your front door turn almost as quickly as employees leave the organization? The manager of today will look beyond its own annoyance with the revolving workers. We need to look at what we are doing to get our workers to leave quickly. In reality, if you lose your professional, experienced staff at any point, it's time to change how you handle your employees.

Another way to track what you and other executives in your company do to meet the needs of both your workers and your organization is to use the Employee Life Cycle template. Use this template as your guide to properly manage and retain your staff.

Phase One-Build a solid foundation: the vision and mission statements of the organization are the center of the design Employee Life Cycle. How do the staff know what is the best decision for business and jobs without a core theme or ideology for every employee? To really make these statements effective, they need to show how you value your employees and treat them. Therefore, every director must take responsibility for all actions to follow up on your mission's employee and corporate focus.

Step Two –Integrate mission: it is important to follow through with the center of your business. Take a look at all forms of interactions, every attempt to inspire you and every aspect of your physical and mental environment, and ask yourself, "Does this represent the intent of your mission?"

Phase three–Comprehending the Employee Life Cycle: The Employee Life Cycle splits into seven doable and workable stages. You will ensure that all the support systems concentrate on attracting and retaining the best employees by mastering each process. Both phases reflect the stages of organizational training and how managers are able to handle workers ' needs best.

Step One-Jobs. This process can be defined as "what you see is what you get," which is what the public sees in you as a future employer when they join you. So you want the public to see how amazing you are in the job process. Your job ads will speak about your culture and explain clearly the roles and expectations for each role. The managers must prepare to perform innovative interviews that analyze the true skills and work ethic of each employee. If your appearance is not appealing, only the amount of workers who are willing to work for a' less than desirable' employer can be attracted.

You and your managers must first have strong criteria on whom to recruit and then create a solid interview and selection process that delves further into the skills and abilities of the candidate so that you can hire the best.

Finish this step with a specific positive picture as to why you can't live without the best candidate! Then recruit them. Recruit them.

Step Two-Orientation: It is important to give that employee a genuine welcome and guidance. You must consider the company as a whole and the goals of the team and the job. Please note that your top candidate has probably received many offers. They're just going to leave if you annoy the new employee. You must be consistent in delivering the picture you conveyed during the interview immediately. A comprehensive, practical approach, which gives them the right tips and resources, will, therefore, pay off.

Step Three learning: whether you are implementing training programs or developing your job skills, let them know that you respect them, and want to grow them into a more strong team member. Education is a very competitive advantage in the labor market today. This is an assumption for new staff. In this region, you should be a chief.

Step Four–Assessment: truthful, timely, and developmental reviews are key to our success. Nevertheless, most managers tend to fail to understand the motivation of each worker to exccl and how direct feedback accelerates success. Assess employees ' efficiency, skills growth, effective learning, and interpersonal skills in a way that will maximize their value for the company. Employees want to learn how and where they are-be them new or seasoned workers. Don't leave them wanting. Don't leave them wanting.

119

Step 5-Reward: evaluation then feedback alone is insufficient. A consistent, meaningful reward system and fair must be applied to it. Rewards should include awards and verbal recognition, and creative and financial rewards to help employees understand how high their contributions are. Create formal and informal award systems that inspire and empower workers. Involve employees in the development of their own compensation systems. The best way to satisfy your wishes is to be honest with your budget constraints but also to ask them what advantages and incentives they want. Maybe you're shocked.

Step Six–Challenge: Many people are motivated more by greater obligations, sharing their skills, choosing tasks, and other organizational challenges. But only those workers who perform at high levels and those employees you want to retain must be spared. Develop ways to improve their careers, reinvigorate them, and reward them with their work and be less likely to seek job satisfaction elsewhere.

Sixth stage: failure to question your staff is one of the most common reasons why your staff is leaving your agency. Nonetheless, like every stage of the Employee Life Cycle, keep professional when you quit the organization. Thank you for your contribution, for performing and using data from exit interviews and tracking and reviewing turnover statistics to help you make better decisions on jobs and administration. Retention: By keeping in touch with your team at every point of your career, you can continue to pursue new tasks requiring additional direction, preparation, assessment, incentives, and challenges. The rate of people spinning out is low as cycling continues. In every step of the Employee Life Cycle, you can do so much to stop the spin cycle. Evaluate how each step of your organization functions. Build staff teams to work in each process so that you are the sort of employer that attracts employees. You may be one of those businesses that do not have such a poor effect on employment rates because your workers do not fall out.

CHAPTER FIVE

Ayurveda's Longevity Secrets

Eternal young people are a subject which has fascinated humanity over the years.

Scientists are now looking for ways to attain eternal youth by observing old age. The mechanisms that contribute to, or induce, aging are referred to as "age markers."

These are some essential indicators:

oxidative stress–pollutants, radiation, stress, and even the metabolism of the body create free radicals that break up other molecules. The body usually mops free radicals, and equilibrium is retained. But if the body can't cope, oxidative stress spreads like the flames, causing quick aging-as a cut apple turns brown and wrinkles.

Inflammation— Pain, redness, swelling, and heat usually occur when the body tries to repair damage and to remove invaders. When we age, the body tends to overreact, get over-inflammatory, and cause diseases such as atherosclerosis, inflammation, allergies, and self-inflammatory conditions-when the body is self-inflamed.

Cell proliferation–Cells are programmed to live die when they are finished. When cells break the rules, they refuse to die. Instead, it can be risky to split into more rogue cells. Typically the body detects and kills rogue cells. When we age, however, our immune system gets affected, and these rogue cells can become cancer.

Lower stress adaptation-Age is marked by reduced stress management skills and their effects-high blood pressure and blood sugar, poor appetite, diminished immunity, and reduced sexual performance.

Finding Solution

The problem of aging has been discussed by the human race for thousands of years. Indian ayurvedic medicine has been dedicated to keeping people healthy so that they can live 100 years or more. And a whole branch of Ayurveda discussed the Rasayana-longevity theory.

The authors of the first Ayurvedic texts praised the youth-preserving virtues of several herbs, including Amalaki, haritaki, ashwagandha, Guduchi, pippali, shilajit, and Shatavari. Jams, wines, tablets, and other life-promoting preparations that are still used today have been prepared with recipes.

Longevity Herbs

Modern research on Rasayana plants has generated interesting results–all of these herbs have antioxidant, anti-inflammatory, anti-cancer, and anti-stress properties combined! They remove the aging signs!

To couples preparing childbirth, pregnant mothers, newborn babies, children, and adults–and for those of their mature years-Ayurveda recommends Rasayana herbs. Practitioners will customize a lifetime Rasayana program to match your gender, type of body, genetic vulnerabilities, and history of health.

Panchakarma It was, however, considered that the body should be purified of toxins for these herbs to work optimally. Just as it is impossible to substitute the oil without maintaining a clean oil filter, the cells of the body will not be able to absorb rejuvenated herbs efficiently without eliminating waste and contaminants trapped beforehand.

Panchakarma is the effective detoxification process of the body by Ayurveda, including (research has found) environmental toxins that have been present in the fatty tissues for dozens of years. Traditionally, panchakarma care is prescribed twice a year at the turn of the season. A Rasayana regimen of rejuvenating plants and a healthy diet follows.

Diet Ayurveda suggests a diet that is easy to digest but nutritious. Most foods are designed to improve digestibility, and raw foods are just a small part of a healthy diet. Spices are used for digestibility enhancement.

Even more important than what you eat is how you feed! For proper digestion and for proper tissue formation, relaxation during meals is necessary, Ayurveda says.

A number of good quality fats, particularly to reduce excessive inflammation, are required for health. We need omega-3 oils to offset not only omega-6 but also too saturated fats.

Eat foods rich in antioxidants, like vivid fruit and vegetables. Using ginger, turmeric, garlic, tamarind, and cinnamon spices. Clove oil is one of the best-recognized antioxidants. Prunes, oranges, grenades, and berries are high in antioxidants.

Ayurvedic nutrition advice requires no rules or contradicts modern nutrition advice; a trained practitioner can assist you in incorporating the information that meets your personal needs and constitution.

LifeStyle of life Manages the pressure to prevent damage caused by free radical development, poor digestion, and a weakened immune system. Understand and use relaxation techniques like yogic breathing every day.

Respiration and relaxation help the body to reach the conditions in which it can heal and stabilize itself. We also increase prana, or coordinate life forces-which enhances strength and the capacity of the body to deal with stress.

Harnessing the mind

Harmonization of the mind Avoids frustration, fear, jealousy, and other negative emotions and feelings. Any bad thought causes a cascade of physical harmful chemicals in the body. Cultivate yourself and transform into more optimistic thoughts and emotions if you want to stay young.

Ayurveda says that disease is often caused by "faulty thinking," muddled thought in which we make healthy choices in terms of diet and lifestyle. Controlling negative thinking provides clarity of mind, in which we take rational health choices.

Physical activity without stress

127

Modern Yoga will consistently help you manage pressure and achieve greater mental clarity and self-awareness. Moderate physical activity, such as Yoga, promotes the body's good functioning, strengthens the immune system, and increases the adaptability of the body to stress. Excessive exercise, however, improves the free development of radicals and degenerative disorders. Ayurveda recommends a slightly higher breathing and sweaty workout.

Act young to stay young

Join young people to Maintain a young attitude. What do kids and young people do most of the time? They're off!
Find ways to become playful and childlike, which will also make the body young. Research shows that young people are less genetic than old people, while they are of the same chronological age.

Realigning with natural rhythms

Relaxation of natural rhythms Eventually, take time to adapt to nature. Being in nature reminds us of the flow of life, the eternal process of creation. When we are once again, part of the natural cycles of growth, we relax and let our bodies function at their best and gracefully mature in their own natural time.

So is true longevity?

"Longevity" means the optimum functioning of the tissues and life processes-throughout our lives. The Ayurvedic and Yoga sciences offer the most comprehensive health-optimizing and slowing aging system possible. I think this provides tremendous potential for human quality of life and needs more study.

No "one-size-fits-all" solution is available. Ayurveda recognizes that everyone has unique needs, and it is therefore recommended to establish a relationship with a trained Ayurvedic practitioner if you take good health and longevity seriously.

Women's Energy Bodies: Making the Most of Your Phases and Life Cycles

The cycles of women's energy bodies were ignored in both traditional and new age spiritual teachings as well as in mainstream and alternative remedies. Bear in mind that I am not a healer, so my main interest is spiritual-how knowledge of, and use of our different energy systems can contribute to our spiritual growth, particularly through experiences that are only available if we have full access to our personal power. These teachings are mainly found in the tradition of Kundalini Yoga and Vajrayana Buddhism, but I have as well found in various shamanic traditions, heathen traditions, medieval Christian female mystics, kabbalah, and soufism.

In general, the energy bodies of women are more flexible, absorbent, and fluid than the bodies of men. Men are denser and more naturally behave like a shield. We, women, are more overwhelmed by energies that can become the energy of intuition, but also a source of dispersion and mental diversion.

Our energy body's tolerance operates in phases that lead to our monthly menstrual cycle. During the first third, which leads to ovulation, our energy body is a little resilient, and we react more externally. They are more sensitive to external forces and often more inward-oriented in the second half leading to menstruation.

Puberty: Swinging, developing, puberty, is the beginning of these monthly cycles. It is a period of intense psycho-spiritual changes, as well as physical changes and intense hormonal (including in the brain). Just as a girl's body becomes a female body, her energy body becomes a female energy body. And the problem with our society is that it is still sexually processed.

Besides being absorbent, our energy bodies are more attractive. We are like small magnets that are drawing on other energies, especially in the first half of our period. This can prevent us from realizing that this power, which is the' yin' component of creation, can be utilized for other purposes, especially the

131

creative ones (and I'm using' creative' in the sense of anything that we want to create in our lives, not merely artistic attempts).

Work on the understanding that procreative power is not only sexual; it is part of your overall personal strength and can be applied to all your creative efforts.

Early Adulthood: Sexuality, game, Cycle Conscience
Hopefully, our late youth, and twenties are a time in which we grow our personal power, learn how to guide our goals by understanding our normal psycho-spiritual cycles. But if we only control our personal power through our attractiveness, we will focus too much on attracting others. This is, to some degree, the case for most of us, and few of us emerge from this time with our full personal power. We are missing the opportunity to gather in a way for the purposes of our wider life, including our religious awareness.

From a spiritual perspective, I think that the best thing we can do is to possess our personal strength during this stage–more precious than explicit spiritual study or practice. And with any

132

event, we feel passionate about and aspire for excellence inside, and we may possess our personal power. With concrete external objectives during this phase, we learn about the ebbs and flows of our energy cycles. That said, it is particularly beneficial to cultivate a meditation practice during this period.

Concentrate on cultivating personal power and manifesting it in reality throughout your life, whether through higher education, job, athletics, the arts, hobbies, or (of course) spirituality.

Childbirth: ride happiness, release/surrender, enjoy the relations with the' other hand' For those who choose children (more about this later), childbirth can be an awe-inspiring time to develop your creative and intuitive skills, (backaches, nausea,). On the other hand, you can feel your the link to' the other side' (I'll leave it ambiguous, like the word ' energy body,' so that I can keep it non-denominational) as if holding a life in you had opened up a door for life to come and now through that door you can also go the other way through.

133

This is a great time to go inside. Meditate, read religious books, pursue natural and artistic desires, and plan for the challenges ahead, of course.

Concentrate on improving intuitive abilities and riding pleasure as part of being more related to the other side.

Motherhood: bearing loads, juggling mother and child energy demands The childbirth ' doorway' opens very rapidly in the first eight weeks, normally after parting. It can be painful in addition to hormonal changes and sleep deprivation. It ensures that some women float through this process of transformation (more power to them). If you have developed spiritual awareness, this period is simpler, because you are able to continue' traveling' on the relaxation rates you learned during childbirth yourself.

Whether you have time or energy to do that is something else! Your energy system actually is now extended to cover your baby (they don't call it the' fourth half,' for nothing) for almost two decades you won't regenerate the energy entirely (and some people never do it). And the same applies to every additional child you have. Motherhood is a sacrifice on an energy level, simple and simple. It's a gesture of love, perhaps. If so, psychologically, it can bring you back as much as you put in.

To do that, you have to make peace with the sacrifice and schedule your energy use and growth. Ideally, in each cycle of development, your children have their own personal strength more and more, and you can take yourself back a little bit. Gradually, it is important to regain this energy and to take care of yourself enough that you are not fully swallowed up, mentally and energetically. This is mostly about spirituality in this process.

Reflect on finding the right energy balance between providing your child with age-specific energy and restoring your personal strength as he or she develops.

Maturity Childfree: Improved collectivity, pursuing advanced instruction The premenopause adult years are a massive spiritual opportunity for women who do not have kids (by default or circumstance). It is very important, I believe, to say this because the moral importance of women in many religious traditions seems to be equated with motherhood. Those who put this forward seem to forget that in all religious traditions, most of the more prominent mystics, male or female, did not have families and in most instances, were celibates.

While many people think that is because of moral reasons, if you read the actual teachings in religious practices, it is clear that the energy benefit of celibacy and/or childlessness was originally recognized. In fact, remaining childless is considered an advantage or even a prerequisite in the complex based energy yoga, like certain lines of Tantric Kundalini and Buddhism yoga, in order to receive advanced instruction, especially for women. Because to perform these practices theoretically, you must have access to 100% of your procreational forces, which these exercises allow you to turn to meditative techniques. A woman who has children has clearly spread too much energy in her life. This isn't to say that we mothers don't attain illumination, spiritual liberation, or

136

anything you want to call it. (Of course, a lot of women did not live past their childbearing years till last century, so maybe more mothers, with adult children who have reactivated their energies fully.) For some parts during our maternity years, it only makes some power strategies and certain directions a challenge. And these specific obstacles are not addressed to childfree women. So the heavens are the limit! Explore your personal power and spirituality of all kinds, especially those based on energy. This energy is also used in spiritual realms, divination, energy healing systems, and the creative arts.

Concentrate on increasing your intuition and energy awareness and turning your procreational energies into the mysterious directions of any spiritual tradition which you share.

Perimenopause: Introduction to Mystic Hood Perimenopause is the introduction to menopause that is biologically 1 to 10 years long (which would be in many women's late 1940s and early fifties). Regrettably, most doctors and health professionals do not even know this stage because the symptoms can be small and fluctuating and because they were initially first and

137

foremost created by men on the basis of an interpretation of men's bodies.

Just as this is a physical transition period with fluctuating signs and symptoms, this is also true on the spiritual and energy levels. Ideally, a mother took her power for herself (or at least she was out of the early days of intense childhood), and a child-free woman studied the spiritual stages of her consciousness. Both are now planning for an entire revival as a mystic during menopause.

The entire period of perimenopausal energy is a preparatory phase. The monthly body energy cycles are starting to dissipate and, when properly prepared, become increasingly more intuitively aware and stronger.

Concentrate on establishing or continuing to develop a practice of meditation and discovering energies and spiritual lessons that appeal to you.

Menopause: Birth of a Mystic: I openly use the term "mystic" to refer to religious seekers and educators who focus on personal and specific divinity encounters. Being a mystic does not require light, but means a certain approach to religion–not a religious one, but a consciousness-based one. Our consciousness is infinite, but our thoughts and emotions and our own sense of self generally weigh down too much to feel them. Generally speaking, metaphysical spirituality is to go outside the human being and to fly through our consciousness to other planes. It requires an extraordinary level of knowledge and power over both our consciousness and our energy system.

We can practice mysticism anytime in our lives, but there are challenges and distractions to do so at every stage of our lives as I have tried to describe it. Ideally, they're all gone at and beyond menopause. If we have our own personal power and our magical knowledge of our consciousness has been established, we can take menopause to the limit when we do not. Most oriental and indigenous cultures identify this process as the most sacred in the life of women. If before that we haven't become a magician, we know time is right.

139

Concentrate on the re-establishment and/or ownership of your

personal power, on expanding your spiritual understanding and

practices.

Human Longevity and Life Expectancy in the Future

This problem is vast and has immense consequences for humanity, both individually and collectively, what it is going to mean for you and how to ensure that you are fully prepared to use the opportunities available to maximize your healthier staff life longer.

THE REVOLUTION OF LONGEVITY I think we are very fortunate to live in such an exciting time as mature people in a developed nation. The Movement for Longevity is almost here and gives hope and hope that we could all looking forward to far longer, healthier lives than we could ever imagine 15 years ago. The breakthrough in longevity has already occurred in biotechnology and medical sciences and will lead to a quantum change in our life span, but more significantly, in how long we will stay healthy, i.e., our "healthspan."

Right now, longevity statistics tell us that the average birth life span for the top 20 countries is 80; on average, however, the last eight years (10 percent) are spent on health problems.

It would be futile, probably unfair, and even more urgent to prolong our life span without enhancing our health status at a time when the increasing population of people over the age of 65 is in danger of swamping them.

HUMAN Lifespan-THE LAST Hundred years Before looking into the crystal ball and looking into the future, let's take a look at the recent longevity history and current life expectancy figures.

"Life expectancy" is really the average number of years for which a person can expect to live if they are experiencing the existing "age-specific" mortality rates in the population, according to the WHO(World Health Organization). In other words, there are no significant changes in a person's life, whether positive or negative.

The life expectancy in developing nations has risen by 50 percent over the last 100 years, compared to 53. Six years to eighty-four years. This was due to a combination of two factors: increasing mortality among children and older people living longer.

"Broken Limits for Life Expectedness" "For 160 years, the highest performance life expectancy has increased steadily by a fourth of a year a year, which is a constant exceptional achievement in humanity."

THE WHY FUTURE TOO FROM HERE?

Many long-term scientists believe that over the next ten years, there will be dramatic advances in biotechnology that will change the future longevity prospects radically, with a significant increase in life expectancy for all of us. It is commonly believed that in developed countries, an average life expectancy of 100 years is possible in that period.

143

Acting in all key areas of your lifestyle right now will increase your chances of benefiting from these eventual advantages.

My research suggests that four fields of ongoing research, growth and public education must be tackled concurrently and urgently if as many of us as possible are to benefit in full: 1. The great work carried out in chronic degenerative diseases by medical institutes, and public medical practitioners worldwide have already saved many lives and improved the lives of many others and need to continue.

2. Continue education of people; the fact that contracting these chronic conditions as they get older is not unavoidable and that they can dramatically reduce the risk of contracting it, i.e., by following a balanced anti-aging diet and avoiding unhealthy foods and ingredients, preventing unhealthy addictions, by regular practice of exercise and fitness and by

3. "The scientific evidence now clearly upholds the notion that it is time to invest in the future of humanity by fostering the necessary political will, public support, and resources needed

144

to slow down aging, and so on. As I said in the introduction, in
biotechnology and medical science, the longevity revolution is
taking place and will put a quantum leap forward in our lives,
but more importantly, how long we remain healthy.
What 20 years ago, science fiction would have been considered
to be a reality. The 2003 human genome project has opened up
a number of exciting possibilities. The field of' tissue
engineering' enables the medical laboratories to build
replacement organs and body parts using their own cells, and
windpipes, breast tissue, new organs, and bladders are already
under production, including many body part of another.

In the next ten years, major biotechnological developments will
dramatically change our future survival prospects, with a
significant increase in the life expectancy of all of us. There is
strong confidence that in developed countries, an average life
expectancy of 100 years is possible in that period.
By acting now in all key areas of your lifestyle, you will
increase your chances to benefit from these imminent benefits
and live much longer, healthier, and happier lives.

145

How to Sustain Longevity on the Court

This chapter will teach you how to play basketball for a longer time. Whether you're going to spend longer in a single or long day, I'm going to discuss important things that can help you achieve that. The topics I'm going to cover are a person's diet, stretching, preparation, and a person's desire to play the game.

Diet To begin stuff, I will discuss the essentials of a man's diet with a brief overview of several forms of supplements that can also aid. What you put in your body ultimately determines how well your body works. You will naturally take a lot of calories if you eat loads of fatty foods and candy. You may think that taking in a lot of calories would help you play basketball for longer, but you're wrong if you think you will do it by eating fatty food. Ultimately, calories supply the body with the fuel needed to perform tasks like exercise, but fat calories are not the healthiest way to get this power. One gram fat contains nine calories, while four calories per gram of protein and carbohydrates are present. When you consume plenty of fatty foods, it can have long-term effects on your skin, which will essentially discourage you from lasting longer. The possible side effect of eating fatty foods is weight gain. Weight gain happens when calories that are not consumed from exercise are retained. Basketball is still possible if you are heavier than normal, but if you are out of form (agility and stamina will affect), you won't be able to last on the court. While weight gain is possible to eat high-protein or carbohydrate foods, you're better able to keep calories from fatty foods. Fatty foods can also increase your cholesterol, which can affect the body's health.

"If a person has too much blood cholesterol in the bloodstream, excesses can be introduced into the arteries, including the coronary arteries in the cardiovascular brain, carotid arteries in the heart, and in those arteries that supply the blood of the legs.

There are many things you may want to include in your diet so that you stay longer. The first may be obvious and quite repetitive, but vegetables are a vital component of your diet. When you eat vegetables frequently and then good for you, it is

147

a good beginning. You can eat at least eight portions of vegetables a day. By taking into account a Clean-energy-ideas.com list of high-energy vegetables (sprouts, asparagus, spinach, and broccoli), green vegetables seem to be a healthy food option.

Another kind of high energy food is fruit, as you may have inferred by the last food mentioned. Sugar, water, protein, and vitamins, b, b1, b2, b6, c, and e are included in the fruits. Fruits provide a large amount of water that supplies the water required to play basketball to your body (which consists of approximately 57 percent of water). Basketball can be a very complex sport, and sweat comes with fatigue. Sweat is used to cool down the body, but also to reduce your body's water. You should first and foremost have some kind of drink nearby to stay hydrated, but eating fruit will help regularly. Fruits also contain a wide variety of vitamins that offer the body a natural boost to immune and stronger. You can't play basketball if you're sick without, of course, eating fruit, you are Michael Jordan (who played with flu in the NBA finals).

Many energy-efficient, healthy foods include nuts, grains, fruit and vegetable juices, eggs, and yogurt. Nuts and seeds are a food type snack that you can quickly eat before playing basketball. Eggs can be in large quantities unhealthy, so you should try to limit your egg consumption, but they are a big protein source.

Protein is a crucial amino acid that the body constantly requires. When you play basketball, you will use different muscles in your body. Protein plays a major role in the reconstruction of muscle tissue that can have an effect on running up and down the court, football, and baseball. Because the body can not store protein for further use, you should regularly consume high-protein foods if you expect to last on the court. Many high-protein foods consist of various kinds of meat, dairy, eggs, and even milk.

As a precautionary measure, relaxing people always tell you to "stretch before physical activity." How many of us do this? I'm going to be the first to tell you that I tend to forget this many times. Anything hypocritical of me, but easy to forget. Most of the time I'll stretch after I played a bit because I'm not going to feel as loose as I want to. Stretching is extended, so even though you fail to do it before you start playing, you should still do that. If you play basketball, given that you use your legs A LOT, you want to stretch every muscle in your body. Keep your stretches for about 10 seconds and keep them in the same place until you are finished. Stretching can reduce both your chances of injury and your soreness after activity, stretching increases mobility and enhances the range of movement of your joints. When you play basketball, the benefits of working out outweigh the costs. It doesn't take much time to make sure that you stretch before playing!

Training You might think basketball training involves practice, shooting, etc. But what I mean by learning is that the body is both cardiovascular and muscular. Basketball involves a lot of heavy breathing and jumping. You demand a lot from your body, and if your body is not in good physical shape, it may be hindered. You can get in shape by running or sprinting to make heavy breathing and fatigue beneficial for your body. After a while, you will spend more time with the wind as you were when you started. Another thing you should remember is to boost your muscle strength. As I said before your feet, a large part of basketball is played. You should start doing various leg exercises, including lunges, squats, and calves, to strengthen your legs.

CHAPTER SIX

Stress and Longevity

Do you want to live forever? That may not be possible, but you certainly want to live your lives with dignity, health, and happiness.

Many people realize that their daily lives can be stressful and can affect their health or, at least, their quality of life. Everyone has growing stressors, and everybody has their own specific way to react to these stressors. Although we are all special, it is very important to realize that being a "victim" of our stressors is practically normal and can be kept to a minimum with education. Stress will and will affect the natural response of our body to aging.

Symptoms like nausea, aches in the mouth, back pain, high blood pressure, abdomen (including discomfort, poor absorption, diarrhea, and constipation) heart rate, breathing, sexual dysfunction (and satisfaction), rates of panic / anxiety, depression, other types of arthritis and most commonly sleep disturbance may cause or worsen stress. Stress could play a role in overall health or worries: the power level, hair, weight, and success levels. The aging process can be exacerbated by excessive stress in negative ways.

Stress can influence your quality of life in subtle ways. Even in the middle of life, we see our energy level getting lower. Perhaps we find that we can't focus as much on activities as we want. These may be less extreme than major painful symptoms, but they can be a way to steal our satisfaction and decrease our productivity! We don't have to be anxiety survivors.

Sensitivity and proper self-care to mitigate the impact of stress will help you reduce the negative effects of the pressure of your life if not. If stress is rising, people live longer, healthier, and happier lives. All possible positive side effects of health and effective stress management include efficiency, innovation, increased energy levels, and an enhanced capacity to interact more clearly.

While bad habits can start in childhood, learning and cultivating positive coping skills that boost your quality of life never gets too late.

Understand the issues: How many of us are overwhelmed by our children's development and their autonomy (and our lack of control over their choices?) How many of us battle aging parents, siblings, and spouses in ways that raise our daily stress? This is because of our concern and love and because we have no influence over the issues of these family members.

We lose some of our strength and flexibility when we are "mature." The stuff we used to "treat" now seems to come to us. We are not as informed as we would like to respond to current issues. Things like: the economy, the war on terrorism, the effect of the press on our children, the situation in our communities all seem to touch us now more than ever before. The degree of change we once expected and welcomed tends to be more daunting as we get older. Fears and anxieties will affect us more and more because we do not have the power, strength, or resilience to change as quickly as we did when we were younger.

Ten tips to reduce the pressure that affects our longevity are available here.

1. Stress management

Daily reflection, with moments of gratitude and appreciation. Techniques of ventilation. Deep relaxation, tolerance, and regulation of physical and emotional stress symptoms. When you begin a daily practice of deep relaxation to reduce pressure, it may take 4-6 weeks to start seeing results. The maximum benefit of this program can require 8-12 weeks of regular daily use. It takes time to change life-long patterns, which encourages you to dream not possible.

2. Exercise

Train at least five days a week in more than 30 minutes to minimize muscle stresses, increase energy, and strengthen your body. (To take into consideration walking, running, jogging, rowing, cycling, escalating, biking, swimming, etc.)

3. Diet / Nutrition

Caffeine elimination. Do not depend on alcohol or drugs to manage stress. Using sufficient supplementation of essential trace minerals and antioxidants (such as chromium, calcium, magnesium, etc.).

4. Planning

Know and work towards your goals. Should not forget to schedule your creative, esthetic and mind needs, social interactions, finances, a career with friends and family, and spiritual needs. Don't stop learning or trying new stuff.

5. Communication

Learn to listen now! Develop the best skills for clarification in your thoughts and feelings and then find the best ways of communicating these thoughts appropriately. When you concentrate on what your partner says, not on your reaction, you will be able to respond more relaxedly and convincingly to questions or objections.

6.Surpport

 No man is an island. If necessary, we need a community of friends and family to support us. Give as much as you get. Give as much. And remember to allow others to give you. (This is hard, but you can deliver the greatest gift!)

7. Spiritual well-being

Know how to connect with your mind and then spend time. Know what brings joy and happiness to you and do these things. Your journey can lead you to a beautiful outdoor venue, or a quiet time in which children can play in a garden or in an art museum or in a park.

8. Avoid negative attitudes.

Avoid negative people and stay in negative thought. Taking good care of yourself and in every experience, find the best. Learn from errors and smile at the lessons, especially when they are difficult.

9. Acceptance

Free from fear and found acceptance what we all have to face. Easier said than done, but you will have the inner strength and love to cultivate acceptance from deep within when your life involves regular self-care. It is amazing what daily stress management can do to help you find peace and acceptance.

10. Humor

Laugh everyday loudly. Create circumstances in which you can smile and laugh with joy and fun. Make a special pleasure hunt!

Keys To Longevity And Youthfulness

Growing old is a normal lifestyle. Nevertheless, this does not mean you will embrace a "normal" progression of aging of diseases like diabetes, heart disease, or cancer.

Scientists urgently need to find ways of preventing aging. But more and more studies show that you can remain healthy and fit through your later years just by changing your diet and lifestyle.

Below are seven strategies that have a significant impact on your longevity and youthfulness.

Optimize insulin levels Insulin is an effective inhibitor of the aging process and has a huge impact on your lifespan.

Insulin is released when you eat carbohydrates to mop up the additional blood sugar that creates carbs. When you eat too much sugar and grain over time, and your body produces an abundance of insulin continuously, your cells become immune. This ensures that to achieve the same results, you need even more insulin. It becomes a vicious cycle.

Most people today have high insulin levels because of our typical sugar-laden diet and sleepy lifestyle. Diabetes is the most well-known disease, but studies show that it could also be osteoporosis, cancer, or cardiovascular disease. At the molecular and cellular levels, the root cause of the problem is always, and insulin plays an essential role.

Research indicates how insulin affects two longevity and youngness genes in your body. More insulin flips on the first gene, which encourages aging and shores life, while the second gene, which gives all the advantages of anti-aging, is not disabled.

It means you won't know what the "elixir" gene can do for you— it enhances compounds that make the skin and proteins that build muscle properly function.
It enables the immune system to fight infection.
Turns off cancer-active genes.
This is exactly the reason why scientists believe that the main culprit of premature aging and premature death is high insulin levels.

Optimizing your insulin levels is, therefore, the key to longevity and youth— don't eat refined white carbs or sugars, particularly foods that contain high fructose. Recent studies show that despite the low glycemic index of fructose, excess fructose intake actually kills your insulin sensitivity and induces plaque in your arteries. I had already changed my stance against agave nectar because it contains over 90% fructose, almost twice the height of an artificial high fructose maize syrup, on the basis of this finding.

Recall the sugar thrives in cancer cells. You are already lowering the risk of cancer by cutting it off from your diet. While whole grains and fruit are good for you, they must be moderately consumed. Be aware that some people are more carbohydrate-sensitive.

Exercise Normal to high health exercise (walking, cycling, swimming, dancing) helps improve insulin sensitivity, lower body fat, reduces the risk of cancer, and improves the health of the brain. Take five days a week for at least 30 minutes of exercise.

In addition, include at least two 30-minute weight training sessions a week. Research shows that by age 70, people, on average, lose 22% of their muscle mass, which may make you vulnerable to fatal falls. Additionally, weight training helps to maintain your abilities and slow down the effects of aging on your brain.

Emotional Health–be positive, find a purpose, manage stress, make friends. It's time to change your outlook and mindset, always looking at a glass-half-empty, negative, gloomy, and depressed one. Your state of mind directly affects how your body handles inflammation, which aids most chronic conditions that kill people prematurely every day.

Research show that people who are happy and positive have a purposeful lifestyle are able to manage pressure in life efficiently and are socially active, have stronger immune systems, and live longer, healthier lives with healthy relationships. People living to 100 or more generally have very positive attitudes; they are unusually bright, active, outgoing, and cheerful. You know how to laugh and have fun too often.

Environmental toxins do not burn. Do not smoke. If that is the case, find a way to leave.
Decrease your intake by purchasing organic products and grass meat from pesticides and chemicals.
Reduce your intake by preventing processed foods of preservatives and additives.

Limit your exposure to all forms of radiation.

Reduce your exposure to household pollutants and chemical products by adding non-toxic substitutes to household cleaners, soaps, personal hygiene products, air fresheners, bug sprays, etc.

Most individuals, including clinicians, are not aware of recent research results regarding the importance of vitamin D. Optimize vitamin D levels. A simple blood test called 25(OH)D will assess your vitamin D levels as vitamin D is so important to your health because it plays a vital role in immunity insulin secretion Blood pressure regulation Rheumatoid arthritis Osteoporosis Cancer Alzheimer's disease. Make sure it's 50-70 ng/ml throughout the year.

At levels below 50 ng/ml, the body becomes chronically hungry as soon as you can or use vitamin D. When levels reach 50 ng/ml, the body can efficiently store vitamin D in fat and muscle tissue.

Since it is very difficult to get enough vitamin D from the diet, you also should consider taking a natural vitamin D3 supplement if you do not get adequate vitamin D from the sun. Studies show that up to 1,000 IU per 25 pounds of body weight per day is healthy for adults. The dose depends on your current vitamin D level, so it is best to take a blood test before you begin your supplementation. Talk with your doctor and check the dosage regularly to ensure that your vitamin D is in the optimal range of 50-70 ng/ml.

Higher Omega-3, Less Omega-6 Modern diets stress the good use of polyunsaturated oils made from corn, cotton, maize, sunflower, and safflower. Such oils are rich in omega-6 fats and very quickly become rancid and trans fat — excessive intake of omega-6 results in inflammation and various chronic conditions.

On the other hand, omega-3 fats are anti-inflammatory and counter the effects of omega-6. Omega-3 fats have shown to have a beneficial effect on the brain, cardiovascular diseases, and other age conditions.

Native Alaskan salmon, sardines, herring, and grass meats such as beef, bison, deer, lamb, and poison are Omega-3's best sources. Be aware, however, that most beef on the market is made from maize and not from wheat.

Get your anti-aging antioxidants from your diet because they are scavengers for free radicals that are related to diseases like cancer, cardiovascular disease, Alzheimer's disease, and Parkinson's disease.

Free radicals are harmful by-products of natural cell metabolism but can be produced in the body due to environmental pressure and emotional stress (pesticides, chemicals, cigarette smoke, etc.).

The body produces certain antioxidants internally as part of the body's defense mechanism to protect against free radicals. Yet contemporary life has put so much pressure on our body that we urgently need external support–from an antioxidant-rich diet.

165

These are examples of high-antioxidant foods— blacksmiths, blueberries, blackberries, raspberries, cranberries-red kindness, black fruits-apples, avocados, cherries, pears, plums, pineapples, kiwis-artichokes, spinach, red chips, sweet potatoes, broccoli grains-oats, walnuts, pistachios, pecans, hazelnuts, and almond spices-turmeric, etc.

Steps to Living a Longer, Healthier Life

Everybody wishes to live as long as possible, but many people are not prepared to live longer, financially, and physically. Longer lives sound really good, but the likelihood of chronic conditions rises with aging, which can make life much harder as you age.

So, would you do to make things a reality longer without compromising the quality of life?

Second, you must understand that well-planned aging takes place. When you read this right now, you deserve to be a small

166

percentage of the future population and to be ready for its future. Most people are not prepared for problems as we age, or rather turn their eyes blind. It is nevertheless necessary to plan for tomorrow, to live today better. Preparation is like money in the bank to help you to live and really enjoy a wonderfully long and healthy life.

Why do you have to brace yourself to live longer? Wear and tear on your body; this is the natural aging process. Research data show that 88 percent of American citizens over the age of 65 suffer from a minimum of one chronic medical condition, and Australian statistics indicate that nearly half of the population over 65 have long-term health conditions. These are the truth, and sadly most people agree that poor health is part of aging, but what if you can avoid many of them?

What is chronic disease? A chronic medical condition, illness, or wellbeing that lasts for more than three months and chronic diseases, as predicted, becomes more common as one lives longer.

Chronic or long-term health problems are not only present suddenly. Such causes are usually the result of other extrinsic conditions and can be clarified through alcohol usage, cigarette use, lack of exercise, unhealthy diet, obesity, avoidance of oral care, and not enough sleep. These are just a few of the most significant contributing factors which can lead to chronic diseases such as chronic arthritis, rheumatoid arthritis, and rheumatism polymyalgia.

Diabetes- muscle loss, Blindness, with breathing difficulties.

You must mainly value your own body to lead a longer and healthier life. There are many levels of respect:
1. If you know Hippocrates, you may have read the quote, "Let food be your medicine and let medicine be your meat." 2. Maintaining an ideal weight is very critical because the pounds you have put on, you are far more likely to develop type 2 diabetes, triglycerides and high cholesterol, coronary artery disease (CAD), high blood pressure, sleep apnea and stroke.

Some people have promoted caloric limitation to the fountain for young people: Research has shown that mice, rats, and apes with extreme caloric restriction display all kinds of mental and physical benefits, including better mental function, reduced articular disease, and even fewer cataract cases.

3. Smoking stops affect every major organ in your body. Smoking stops Whether you give up your addiction or never begin it, you're more likely to stay healthier and avoid diseases such as diabetes, lung disease, and heart problems.

4. Remain active or risk it. Remain active. Remain active by walking, biking, gardening, bowling, light lifts, or using resistance bands that are my favorite home workout for any age or fitness level 5. A National Institute of Neurological Disorders and Stroke report showed at least 40 million Americans suffer from chronic, long-term sleep disorders. The effects of sleep deprivation on your body may include the development of diabetes. The study shows that sleep deterioration is related to blood glucose regulation deterioration in type 2 diabetics.

A poor memory, a weight gain, low concentration, and a higher incidence of heart disease (coronary artery calcification) also caused a sleep of 5 hours or less.

6. UV rays not only damage the skin and causing skin wrinkling but are also responsible for an extremely dangerous and deadly form of cancer known as melanoma.

7. Maintaining good oral health–Floss Daily studies have shown that poor oral hygiene goes beyond dental and gum disease, which can cause heart disease, osteoporosis, respiratory issues, and a clear correlation to diabetes.

8. Learn how to de-stress your life A little stress is good for you, since it serves as a little in the brain reminder, but when it goes on for long periods, stress becomes very dangerous and can increase your chances of growth, heart disease, high blood sugar, high cholesterol and increase your risk of depression.

Learn how to de-stress meditation, listen to music, create a diary, have a hobby, and learn how to imagine and think positively.

9. The modern diets are killing us. Take antioxidant supplements. For a thousand years, we have periodically limited our calories and consumed a rich antioxidant diet to constantly consume highly processed foods at low antioxidant levels in the last century. Basically, what this means is that we have more free radicals and pathogens than ever before.

Everyone should take multiple vitamins every day, especially if they eat fast food during the week. Already, you probably heard of supplements by now a vitamin called Resveratrol. It provides the amazing health benefits of red vines and is one of the most potent antioxidants found in red wine or the skin of a certain grape that has been processed into red wine.
The health benefits are quite spectacular: prevention of cancer and longevity are two that are outstanding scientists and propel further work. Studies show that this strong anti-aging

171

antioxidant can protect the heart, prevent strokes, reduce cholesterol, and much more.

Hypnosis

Relaxation is a key factor for longer and healthier life. You can learn how to relax with hypnosis, how to sleep better, and using phobia hypnosis allows you to let go of the fear, which can lead to stress and chronic diseases.

The Power of Enzymes- For Digestion, Nutrient Absorption, and Longevity

Using or bolting the incorrect foods will lead to body reactions, including excess acid and gas, grogginess, and bloating. Are you often in need of antacid after eating certain foods? Whether you know what I'm referring to here, most likely, the problem is that you consume a highly processed or fried diet.

Every type of food is indigestible and can not be easily processed by your skin. Indigestible foods are foods that have lost all their natural enzymes and other essential nutrients. The absence of food enzymes is also called denatured meat. Enzymes are responsible for fruit ripening, spoiling, and redness. Do you still think how not margarine spoils or rots? There are no enzymes available, indigestible, not good for you.

Enzymes were the catalysts needed in the body for safe chemical reactions. Enzymes are protein-based substances that bind with other nutrients that change the body by speeding up tasks such as the digestion of food, nutrient absorption, and tissue maintenance and repair. There are over 2,000 different enzymes involved in the digestion and many other essential bodily functions.

Enzymes function in perfect coordination with other nutrients known as co-factors such as vitamins, minerals, fatty acids, and plant chemicals.
The optimal complex of nature requires the participation or play of all the other team players. This can be the main reason why supplementing or adding various other nutrients alone with artificial vitamins and not whole food vitamins do not work. Without the others, no single element will be the only

magic bullet. It is more complex than that. There is, therefore, no activity of enzymes without co-factors.

The average modern diet consists of too many dried, inadequate nutrients, and cooked foods. Heating any food above 118 ° F kills enzymes and other important natural nutrients. A good rule to follow in order to obtain more enzymes is raw vegetables, steamed before they are cooked, poached before hard-boiled, and meats that are rare before they are well boiled.

Some experts believe 80% of our energy is used to digest a typical meal for cooked and processed food. Our burdened digestive system operates 24/7 to break down food that is mostly indigestible or only partly digestible. It could take days or never to remove a meal!

Thanks to this ongoing process, just around 20% of the body's power remains for other important functions, such as thought, breathing, seeing, and helping the immune system, to name only a few. It's like that... You have to free up more of the digestive and digestion cycle if you want to stay healthy or get better.

Whether you eat white sugar and flour, trans fats, or any other undigested product, the body tries to break it down with enzymes. Foods that are easy to digest and eliminate on your body are organic, raw, or lightly cooked. When producing enough digestive enzyme jus, your body won't have to waste energy to turn food into a half-usable form.

Most modern societies consume a lot of non-foods, never intended to create a healthy body. We recognize that over the years, we have not evolved as animals that eat burgers, fries, pizzas, sodas, and beer. Such chemical bombshells literally can not be broken down by our digestive system. That material is not properly digested, and it will only be placed into the intestines indefinitely without enzyme activity.

Some of these escapes into the bloodstream from the intestines and the whole body. Body organs that were never supposed to remove toxins just try to do that. Organs such as kidneys, lungs,

175

and skin can become inflamed and diseased by the poor diet and insufficient digestive system to eliminate harmful residues — the tragic effect on cooked whole food or fast-food diets.

To choose to eat healthier deliberately includes eating more food as raw or lightly cooked as possible. In order to help the body in a more efficient digestion and elimination cycle, consider eating at least one meal a day.

Ideally, we would eat 80 percent of our food this way, but most of us will sadly most likely not. What can you do to help promote this important process in your body and extract possibly large amounts of bonded body sludge?

In fact, you make a wise decision to boost your overall health by adding a decent digestive enzyme supplement to any nearby health food store.

All of us, from the elderly to small children, will benefit from this special knowledge. We will put what is not in our food back. It is much better than using a local medical practitioner who never learned much about enzymes in medical school, rather than coping with diseases by masking opioid effects.

Seek a full complement of enzymes that will split the four main components of the diet: 1.fats / Lipase 2.protein / Protase 3.carbohydrate / Amylase 4.cellulose or cellulase Remember to look for the suffix "ase," which is addressed under the name of the enzyme which destroys the particular element.

Enzyme sources are an easy solution to a range of health problems. If you had a doctor who told you that your diet actually hurts you and damages your health, would it make sense then, if only you knew how the right food and drink could improve your physical condition? Don't count on the majority of doctors to know how to use medicines, operations, and other intrusive measures.

Which solvent is the ideal component of nature to wash and absorb nutrients, and bring no harmful build-up within you? Why, of course, nothing more than rain!

177

CHAPTER SEVEN

The Machine Principle of Longevity

We use everyday machines to make our work easier, to make our lives more enjoyable, but we don't know the parallels between machines and our bodies. We are used to performing the tasks that we consider necessary to achieve our goals, and while we have not built our bodies as we designed our computers, they are similar in the sense that neither can be changed completely but can be updated, adjusted, and enhanced.

The theory of machine derives its core concepts from the obvious connections among machines and the human body. Such principles act as guidelines for people to change their minds, from "I am my body" to "My body is an instrument of my intent." Although it won't dig into your "why," it will help you turn your body into a strong body by providing proper treatment, maintenance, and overall improvement.

Strength: a lower-powered body restricts your strength and is prone to injury in real-world situations.

Conditioning: Gasification is dangerous (and sometimes pathetic) at the wrong time.

Movement: A body not working correctly is malfunctioning or will malfunction due to improper use.

Joint mobility: Proper lubricating of your joints avoids injuries and prolongs the body's functional life.

Lifespan: Efficient training with precise shape is important for optimal performance; repetitive exercises can reduce the body's lifespan.

Nutrition: Your body needs proper fuel to perform optimally.

Power Have you ever driven a car with insufficient power? Going up a steep path is painful; it's a pain on the butt, and trying to get on the highway is frightening. It can change your entire life, both physically and emotionally, rather than simply enhance your sport, career, and outdoor hobbies. How much better would your car feel if you knew that you had another 300 horsepower under the hood? You may never use this power (although you definitely would know how if you followed all the principles), but with every step you took, you gained a lot more confidence. Power and energy are passed to every aspect of your life in your system. This is how the system philosophy approaches the strength concept: incremental strength: you can increase your strength by increasing your workout. Although many ways to do this exist, the main strategies focused on incremental strength are: adding weight, adding members, or increasing difficulty in exercising.

Complex power: from every angle, you need energy. You are not a professional machine; you have one thousand tasks and must be good enough for all of them. You must, therefore, adjust the angles of your movements, which reach the large muscle groups more than just them. It is fantastic to lift thousands of pounds of squatting and jumping, but what about going side by side?

Programmed strength: The Machine Theory integrates the physiological effects of muscle remembering (consolidating a particular task into memory by repetition) over and above "living a healthy life." Studies showed that training in strength helps to improve the interaction between the nervous system and the muscles used, and also showed that strength is affected by internal neural circuits AND external changes in muscle size. Programmed endurance requires collections of specific movements and exercises performed over at least two weeks before development.

Resistance training methods: While the strength theory can be extended to almost all the training methods, Kettlebell training and bodyweight training are the main focus of the system definition. With kettlebell and bodyweight workout plans, the elements of progressive, adaptive, and programmed strength can easily be applied, reduce equipment needs, integrate hundreds of movements, and optimize gains in the shortest amount of time.

Package If you have an older laptop at all, you know what pain a short-lived battery might have in the butt. The battery holds so little energy that you fear that the machine will stop when you move from the living room to the bedroom. The whole thing about having a laptop or a desktop is freedom of movement, so this computer is useless because it can not move even a little. When you treat your body like a machine, make sure it has enough juice to do the job. Just like a laptop with a bad battery, what's right if you can't do your job because the conditioning rate is too low?

For athletes and warriors, you lose the match by running out of steam. Gassing out at the wrong moment could mean you (or someone else) will die for law enforcement personnel, firefighters, and soldiers. Less risky (but Far more pathetic) is someone so out of shape that they may worry about having a break if they park too far away. And, to improve the level of conditioning in your body, the Machine Principles obey those guidelines: intense exercise: you can easily increase stamina without too much strain on your joint by concentrating on short bursts of extensive training. Sets are typically paced, and the exercise is generally performed in a concentrated conditioning span of 20-35 minutes, while additional concentrated conditioning can take up to 4 minutes.

Limited sustainability: While short sprints can give you most of the desired improvements in the fitness you want, limited sustainability will prepare you for real-life situations that require long-term physical effort. Limited sustainability is a key factor. This concept has something to do with muscle strength or the ability of a muscle or a muscle group to sustain repeated resistance contractions for a long time. This is done with high-performance movements such as the Thrust, Snatch, High Pull, Clean & Push Press, and Clean & Jerk.

Weak area conditions: Identifying weaknesses and strengths is critical, and then conditioning accordingly. Exercises to improve endurance and muscle durability in the muscles of the lower leg and feet, muscle corset (core control), hip muscles, and neck and shoulder muscles should be a good fitness exercise. It should also use exercises for relaxing and extending stressed muscle groups, concentrating on hip flexors and external rotors, plantar bending systems and shoulder girdle raises, and forward tilters.

Respiration: regular breathing is a key part of the whole of your body's recovery, which contributes to an isolated release of over-active muscle groups and maximizes effort while increasing your conditioning rate. A lot of oxygen can be produced through the respiration of your stomach (diaphragmatic respiration). Deep breathing improves body relaxation and oxygenation while enhancing conditioning.

Movement Millions of parts, precise technology, and complex equations are used by costly wristwatches to keep track of years, months, hours, minutes, seconds, and a great deal more, with no electronics. You do this by exacting gear movements and other mechanisms. The human body is even more complex than these sophisticated devices. It consists of thousands of moving parts, all of which work together to help you survive and grow when used properly.

Proper movement is an underrated term of dance and martial arts outside. Movement is the intrinsic of action for such people; the energy, conditioning, and physics that go hand in hand are simply by-products. Right movements cause the human body to do awesome things, and wrong movements contribute to dysfunction and injury. The Machine Theory describes motion as follows: Multi-Joint Movements: as you look at traditional strength and conditioning programs, you find they are heavy on single joint, muscle-specific, and single plane movements. Unfortunately, these systems do not adequately represent the everyday needs of a specific sport or functional activity. The system theory uses movements involving a variety of muscle groups that involve movement on several levels. Six-Count Burpee is an example. The movement includes core muscles, head, back, shoulders, and legs and tests your strength, stability, and agility overall. During each phase of exercise learning, multi-joint movements are used in strength and conditioning practice.

185

Multi-planar movements: Multi-planar movements include activities that move the body on one of three moving levels: sagittal (front to back), frontier (side to side), and transverse (turning). Multi-planar movement: The transverse plane is the toughest and most susceptible to injury. Too often, in the first two planes, we overwork our muscles, which limits our functional force and movements and makes us susceptible to injury, often with the lower back. The Multi-planar movement is used in strength and conditioning practice both during that part of the learning with the system concept.

Proper exercise movement: Like a computer, the incorrect alignment will cause extra wear and tear, limited capacity, and sometimes complete failure. For the Machine Theory, the right method for bodyweight and kettlebell practice is important. You can't progress very far without proper form. For instance, when you can do a Barbell Clean improperly at workouts (You know from the hurts on your shoulder and forearm that you're doing wrong), you can not: 1) increase the weight, or 2) increase the difficulty of the workout by adjusting the grip.

186

Proper training movement is discussed by progressions in the exercise complexity by the system theory. For the Clean, you'd start from the ground with the Clean, then a Hang Clean, and then a regular Clean. -variation teaches good movement (for the Clean, -variation reinforces a straight back, strong core, and a tight yanking motion).

Balanced movement: you can't expect to improve your performance without proper balance. Have you ever been through and attempted to find your way through a pitch-black room? It was not just hard because you could not see things in your direction, because you needed knowledge about your body parts and their relationship to each other and your surroundings. It was not easy. By focusing on improving the balance, you do the same with your training. The Machine Theory is intended for controlled movement with a balanced body and kettlebell exercises such as handcuffs, frog stands, one-legged turns, and handguns. Nevertheless, improved balance will also lead to increased efficiency, and in particular, strength and conditioning in all other aspects of the machine theory.

187

You've seen the advertisements where industrial robots with multi-linked arms place doors on vehicles, paint exterior, and welding frames. How would any of this be possible without properly grated joints? Each movement they make, like our bodies, depends on proper flexibility. Despite proper joint mobility, devices (and our bodies) slowly wear off each component until the component has eventually been replaced.

While all principles are applicable to everyone, the Joint Mobility Concept applies particularly for older people who are most vulnerable to injustices due to inadequate mobility. Like an industrial robot, what do you think is cheaper: proper maintenance and repair or replacement of broken parts unnecessarily? The Machine Theory encompasses the idea of joint mobility with basic joint mobility: each joint must be separated and operated independently in several ways. You will always take care of the full range of motions of each joint; this will help prevent tightening and shortening of the muscles and prevent adhesions that can develop across the ligament or tissue, which restricts the flexibility of the joint. Muscle spasticity (contraction), in reaction to increased resistance, can occur and interfere with movement. You want to integrate anatomical motion planes while moving through your range of movement. It includes the sagittal plane (divides the body into two longitudinal parts), the front plane (divides the body into two halves), and the transversal plane. You can improve joint mobility, flexibility, and strength of muscles and joints by carrying out a variety of motion exercises.

Effective Joint Mobility: Joint mobility exercises must be carried out (at least) every day. Joint flexibility exercises include twists, flips, stretches, and a variety of emotions from the neck to your feet. If a particular joint has a problem (stretched and stable brakes are a common problem), the joint must be tested extensively for a long time or a large number of repetitions (100+). Common joint mobility requires at least 10 minutes per day of non-workout and 20 minutes on days of workout.

Longevity High-speed boats, vehicles, and aircraft rely on crazy quantities of energy, precise technology, and huge amounts of money. Highly trained experts develop, check, and

189

maintain them so that they can perform to the highest level when race day arrives. Do you think these million-dollar machines run excessively with little regard to breakage during this process? How, do you think they plan, strategize and check them to ensure without justification that they don't waste time and money?

Most people who need high levels of physical activity (such as athletes, police, soldiers, etc.) feel that they can run unnecessarily on a daily basis, using outdated and unhealthy training methods and proceed on a day of the game and then (some even ignore the future for what they think are now worthwhile benefits. Unfortunately, such people have

Treating the body like a computer ensures that you change it correctly and boost the body durability using the most efficient methods. Would you think it would be better to have a race car lap time just because it had 10,000 laps? Or is it going to improve because it has been correctly tuned and guided to optimize its resources (i.e., power, stamina, and handling)? Long life: proper training and food preparation will enhance the quality of your bones, muscles, inner bodies, and your ability to improve health through diet and exercise. Workout schedules must be based on specific goals (you can't do it all at once) and must continue at least four weeks at a time. We need to take into account the existing level of skills and integrate the various principles in the system theory (no simple task!). Luckily, this concern contains the first-ever machine-compliant workout plan.

Longevity rest and recovery: rest and recovery are as critical as exercise. The entire system will collapse if you follow all other objectives of the machine theory (especially strength and conditioning), but do not include rest and recovery in your routine. Longevity Rest and Recovery consist of 3-on, 1-off, and 2-on, 1-off work schedule, a minimum sleep time of 7.5 hours at night, proper nutrition and medication, as well as cycles of daily cognitive stimulation (e.g., meditation, Holosync, muscle movement relaxation, etc.).

Longevity Tracking: you can't know where you are going unless you remember where you were. Workouts and diet

191

journals do more than just keep you accountable; they provide an accurate record of what was working (and not working), ensure the correct weight, rest, and progression of difficulty and allow you to develop new goals based on past experience. Make sure that you record each set, workout, number of reps/time, weight used, and rest period for workouts. Take care, for food, to document how long you eat, what you consumed, and how much you drank.

Longevity performance testing: It is important to test yourself each quarter (more often than not, and you can block your body and throw out your workout plans) to see whether your exercise and diet works. Longevity quality monitoring is divided into three groups and should be done within 72 hours. Power training, strength testing, and agility testing are categories. To find out more about training and average test results, go to MyMadMethods.com.

Nutrition Rockets contain highly volatile, specially engineered fuels that liberate the Earth from gravity. These special fuels are designed to maximize thrust and also to fit into a rocket without adding much weight or taking up too much space. Likewise, your body needs nutrient fuel to optimize its performance. Note the word "gas," since food should be taken 95% of the time.

Necessary nourishment: if the only aim of a rocket was to provide people with entertainment and fun, cookie dough would be rushed off so the launch pad and the surrounding area could smell like freshly baked cookies. Yet they serve a much larger purpose instead, so they don't. If you were to smile only with food, all food would consist of fat and sugar. Treating the body as a computer means giving it what it needs to do: nutrients in the form of whole foods and supplements if necessary.

Personalized nutrition: there are a number of questions to respond to when you plan your diet, such as: what you like, where you live, food allergies, medical problems, etc. The two fundamental questions that can help to simplify the process are: "What is your aim?" and "How quickly do you want to get there?" Those two simple questions can decide what you eat, eat, and eat.

Consistent nutrition: It is better to adhere to a strict regime for at least three weeks before making changes and modifications. Improvement of your quality is a mixture of appropriate physical, mental, and nutritional concepts. In this way, food starts much earlier than most people realize. In reality, preparation will not be 100% without proper daily food, energy levels will drop, and recovery will take longer.

Water intake for food: Water is important for proper nutrition, as reported by millions of people. At least half of your body weight must be processed in ounces (more days of workout). You also have to drink water on a consistent basis; you must drink a half-gallon of water before or after your workout.

Approaching a problem with a perception

There are five fundamental areas that affect your health. The following are the essential areas to assess your progress. In other words, it will be your "Longevity Road Map."

Stress

 Nutrition

Mindset

Relaxation STRESS Stress is an individual problem. Stress management Approaching a question with a sense of what is unpleasant is special. Many people try to overcome a difficult situation and move on, while others remain there and allow it to settle like wrath. These are the people who are most affected. This will have severe side effects on cardiac, respiratory, circulatory, and immune system health problems. In some situations, the outcome can be tragic because they believe that suicide is the only response. It was understood that holiday seasons and winter months were a very stressful time for many people. The environment will trigger a "cabin fever" to the coop and will wreak havoc with the "circadian rhythm" of the body. This is the internal clock of the body 24 hours a day. This becomes more serious when the local family and friends have no love and support. Loneliness is very tangible and can be almost sliced with a knife.

A study conducted by the National Institutes before 9-11-2001 indicates that stress, anxiety, and mild depression affect almost 50 million people all alone in the US. Unfortunately, the days were even more difficult after 9-11 with the ongoing threat of terrorism. Anyone old enough need only thinks about past events in order to invoke memories that may have slept over the years. Stress is how we respond to a physical or emotional condition or what one sees as stressful. In this stress, the way we react can be either positive or negative. Our reactions will lead to certain situations. In some cases, when we face a challenge, we choose to fight, and in others, we run. With such obstacles, the body reacts by releasing cortisol and adrenaline and decides your course of action with your stress anxiety threshold. In certain cases, constructive reinforcement can help to enable people to deal with a particular task and to achieve the task to their satisfaction. Once the mission is over, you can relax and be glad to have done so. In other words, it's a good job. For some individuals, they need to be anxious to complete this mission.

Negative stress is when a person can not cope with the situation. It will prevent the person from performing a task to their satisfaction under these circumstances. Relaxation is impossible under this scenario, and the individual becomes fidgety and distracted. When this occurs, the health and well-being of individuals will suffer. The end result will be reflected in a range of physical conditions due to a compromised immune system. The preservation of physical and mental health is a problem each person will have to know since there are different circumstances in each case. The evaluation of your stressful situations would be a starting point. You must know the things that set you apart. Recognize symptoms like tight muscles, teeth clenching, and wrathfulness. You will start dealing with anxiety when you learn to listen to what your body is trying to say to you. The body reacts to pressure in three physiological stages: step 1: All cells, tissues, muscles, and organs have an increased demand for glucose. Glucose is

197

required to supply the energy needed for the sudden workload demands of the body. Phase 2: If the workload on the body remains long-term, the rise in glucose occurring in phase one will begin to decrease. As this happens, the body reaches stage three. Phase 3: As in phase two, the brain senses the decrease in the amount of glucose, the body releases cortisone, thyroxine and growth hormone which causes the body to use its resources to produce energy.

This retains glucose at levels that are adequate for the brain and central nervous system to function without them. The battle against stress is a multidimensional program that the patient must also concentrate on himself or herself. These are some tips to support those who feel overwhelming, whatever their cause or type. The number one goal is to have a healthy body and mind. Take the time to relax and practice simple techniques for relaxation. These calming strategies increase your heart rate, reduce your blood pressure, avoid headaches, and prevent abnormally tense muscles.

Start with the basic deep breathing technique slowly and deeply. This can be done whether sitting or standing. Place your hands on your abdomen comfortably. Slowly inhale through your nose. You'll feel your belly growing. Hold your breath for a couple of seconds and then slowly exhale as you whistle your mouth. You're going to feel your stomach deflating. At least 3 or 4 times during each session, repeat this exercise.

Visualization is another method to apply to your relaxation routine. You will use creativity in this technique. Have we not all wanted to be elsewhere? You will do just that with this technique. Free your mind from all foreign thoughts and just let it go. Do you like mountains, sea, hiking, biking, boating, anywhere and all, just let your mind go. Enable 10 to 15 minutes of quiet time to spend your mental holidays. When stress affects a human, the muscles become tight. The extension can be one of the easiest ways to overcome stress. You need to stretch the whole body, starting with your neck, arms, shoulders, upper back, and legs. Stretching while sitting and standing can be achieved. Begin by tilting your head to the right, then a count of 12 to the left. Position your hands, raise your arms upwards, hold 12 and down slowly with the palms up.

First, push the top and bottom further. The best way to do this is to sit down. Sit flat on the floor and slightly spread out on the bottom of the chair with legs. Enable your arms to fall between your legs and slowly lower your body as far as you can without straining. At the lowest relaxed level, in a springlike step for a count of 12, move the shoulders up and down.

You should stretch the upper body while sitting. This can be done while standing, as well. Raise an overhead arm and turn the body with a lower arm to the left. Repeat a count of 6 then end with the process reversed, tilting on the other side.

The next and last stretch is the feet. Lean on, keep your back straight and try to reach your toes as much as you can. You don't really need to touch the feet. Repeat and straighten for a count of 6. Bring the other leg to the line.

Exercise can be a powerful force in your system of relaxation. More about exercise is discussed in the exercise chapter below. Try to find time alone every day for a bit. It would be very helpful to use the visualization techniques listed above at this time. Hearing soothing music is also extremely helpful. Prayers can also offer a troubled soul, happiness, and harmony.

Good night sleep should be a priority number one. It means seven to eight hours of restful sleep. The body's immune system can not cope without adequate rest and is more susceptible to disease.

Recall that laughter can be an infectious power, giving the immune system a boost. The robust laughter, the more advantages you derive.

Allow your responses to others more personal. Go out for lunch or dinner with a friend or neighbor. Use your local community center to meet and socialize with other people.

Do not hesitate to speak to a trusted friend about your pressure issue. Their imputation should prove very beneficial so that they don't hesitate to open it to them.

Mind you're just what you're eating. Don't launch a food binge when distressed. Eat a balanced nutritious diet. Do not pig on junk foods that add huge amounts of calories without the requisite minerals and vitamins. In the food page, more will be covered.

Ultimately, remove alcohol and caffeine. You will restrict alcohol to one drink if you drink, men to two drinks daily. Coffee should not exceed two cups per day. Because particularly if you smoke-STOP!

Antioxidants of Disease Prevention For Longevity

These four most frequently reported causes of death in America to include not drunk drivers, violent shootings, Hiv or illegal drugs, but Heart disease Cancer Stroke Chronically lower American respiratory conditions spent more than $7,400 on health care for the population in 2007, the highest in the world, but our life expectancy is at $45. Japan, by comparison, has invested less than 40% of our jobs, but life expectancy is the world's third-largest!

Despite Americans spending more on health care, the death rates of these chronic diseases continue to rise. The data shows that less processed food and more natural foods are consumed in countries with fewer diseases and longer service life.

Research studies have also shown that almost all of these chronic diseases can be avoided easily by modifying diets and behaviors.

With the amount of processed food that Americans frequently (and definitely more than Japanese) consume, do we deprive our bodies of certain natural nutrients that may help us prevent these chronic diseases?

There has recently been much discussion of the benefits of antioxidants. Below are antioxidants and their function in human health and disease prevention. We will also address whether it is a diet or a supplement to get your antioxidant nutrients.

What causes aging and illness?

More and more medical researchers have found that oxidation induces cell damage and aging.

Oxidation is a chemical reaction in which two or more compounds interact, and at least one electron is lost. Sources of oxidation include a freshly cut apple that turns red, a rusty cycle pan, or a copper penny that turns green.

Stress, prolonged sun exposure, environmental contaminants, cigarette smoke, alcohol, and unhealthy processed foods cause oxidation within the skin.

Oxidation produces highly unstable and reactive free radicals. Free radicals are atoms with unpaired electrons; they target their electron by the nearest stable molecule (with paired electrons). When the targeted molecule loses its electron, it transforms into a free radical itself and therefore causes a chain reaction. The process will cascade and trigger cell damage once it is started.

Your whole body, including your Genes, is constantly being attacked everyday by free radicals. Excessive oxidation weakens the immune system, speeds up the aging process, and is associated with diseases like Alzheimer's diseases, asthma, most forms of cancer, diabetes, illnesses (age-related macular degeneration, cataracts, glaucoma).

Because nature is always able to take care of itself, researchers have found that antioxidants work beneficially against free radicals: antioxidants inhibit the oxidation process by binding to free radicals and neutralizing their harmful effects and thus disrupt its destructive cellular reactions.

Antioxidants scavenge and kill the initiating radicals before oxidation is triggered. Therefore, when you have enough antioxidants to combat free radicals, the body can postpone aging and prevent diseases from harmful free radicals.

As stated earlier, antioxidants are nutrients that prevent oxidation; they bind and stabilize free radicals. Many antioxidants such as catalase, glutathione peroxidase, and superoxide dismutase exist within the skin, whilst other substances must be extracted from the diet. The following are some of the most widely known antioxidants and their health benefits: Alpha-lipoic acid (ALA) is present in red meats, liver, and brewer yeast. ALA is a strong antioxidant that contributes to the regulation of blood sugar and cholesterol levels, decreases inflammation, detoxifies the heavy metal body, and enhances the immune system. ALA can also regenerate other antioxidants such as C, E, glutathione, and Q10 coenzyme. Therefore, if your body has used these antioxidants, it helps to restore them if there is ALA around.

The primary pigments are responsible for the red, orange, yellow & green colors of fruit and vegetables (e.g., beta-carotene, lutein, lycopene, and zeaxanthin). Carotenoids are used to avoid blindness at night, cataracts, macular degeneration, improve immunity, protect against cancer, encourage cardiovascular health, and alleviate both osteoarthritis and osteoarthritis symptoms.

For meats, fish and vegetable oils, coenzyme Q10 (CoQ10) or ubiquinone is mostly made by the liver. CoQ10 has shown its value for congestive cardiac disease, Parkinson's disease, arthritis, muscle weakness, chronic fatigue syndrome, AZT / AIDS therapy, and type II diabetes. CoQ10 improves cardiovascular endurance and increases energy levels.

Flavonoids are a rich compound in fruits and vegetables (e.g., blueberry, ginger, onion, tea). Flavonoids have anti-bacterial, anti-viral, anti-tumoral, anti-carcinogenic, and anti-inflammatory activity. These can also expand the blood vessels, and blood clots can be avoided.

Glutathione Peroxidase (GSH) is the most important natural antioxidant in the body and is synthesized in the cells of the body. GSH protects the vision, boosts the immune system, aids in the transformation of carbohydrates into energy, and prevents oxidized fats from growing in arteries. When detoxifying contaminants such as alcohol, pesticides, or narcotics, it also plays an important role.

Resveratrol is an anti-inflammatory agent present in red grapes and peanuts ' roots, leaves, and skins. Because of the fermentation process, there is much more resveratrol in a glass of red wine than a bottle of grape juice or some of the peanuts. Resveratrol helps prevent blood clots through the widening and stretching of blood vessels, which reduces the risk of cardiovascular disease. It also discourages tumor growth and colon cancer production.

Vitamin C, also known as ascorbic acid, is one of the most active and well-known antioxidants, found abundantly in fruits and vegetables. This helps preserve healthy collagen in body, promote healthy bones and teeth, repair damaged tissue, and improve the immune system. Vitamin C acts as an anti-inflammatory agent and helps the body absorb calcium. It prevents unregulated, pollution-and smoke-causing radical formation and helps recycle oxidized vitamin E.

The main oxidation protector is vitamin E or alpha-tocopherol. Nuts, seeds, and vegetable oils are the best sources. This strengthens the immune system of the body, helps relieve breathing problems, decreases the risk of heart disease, different types of cancer and cataracts, delays the development of certain neurological diseases, and is anti-inflammatory. Vitamin E recycles vitamin C oxidized, and beta carotene oxidized.

The best way to increase our antioxidant levels is to eat a diet high in antioxidants. The body absorbs antioxidants best in food, and the chance of an overdose is very low. The following are six food groups rich in antioxidants, and the examples given are the ones with the most antioxidants in each of the food groups: fruit: Apricot, Apple, berries, avocado, grapefruit.

Legumes: red kidney bean, Black bean, pinto bean.

 Hazelnut, sunflower seed, cocoa, pecan, peanut, walnut.

Spices: Cinnamon, Cinnamon, oregano, tumor.

Tea: White tea, followed by green tea and black tea, has the most antioxidants.

Food: artichoke, cabbage, broccoli, garlic, kale, onion, petty pepper, squash, dark beets, red chocolate, spinach, tomato.

Do we need additional supplements?

209

Although your diet is an ideal source of nutrients, supplements have become increasingly important in contemporary times for three reasons: American diet is high in refined foodstuffs and low in whole organic nutrients.

Urban lifestyles, stresses, and toxins have contributed to the need for additional nutrients.

Intensive practices in monoculture farming have depleted nutrient soil. Research has shown that today's foods have fewer nutrients than those of fruit and vegetables 50 years ago, making supplements a key component of a healthy diet. Nevertheless, it is not advisable to take either one or two mega doses of antioxidants in the case of antioxidant supplements. This is because antioxidant combinations work together as a balanced symphony. Vitamin C and glutathione, for example, recycle oxidized vitamin E while vitamin E recycles oxidized vitamin C and beta-carotene. The trick is, therefore, not the quantity but the mixture. The entire range of antioxidants works together in a loop to defend against free radicals of all kinds. Both these can not be achieved by any antioxidant. While it is unclear whether mega doses of a single antioxidant supplement are truly harmful, it is reasonable to take none alone. Therefore, if you choose to use supplements, you can consult a qualified healthcare professional with the correct combination of antioxidants.

Last but not least, a lot of so-called "superfoods" are now on the market. Some of these superfoods are processed foods with nutritional advantages or disease prevention. Read the labels carefully and be careful about other harmful ingredients such as sugar and additives.

Remember that superfood is not a substitute for "real" food. The organic, healthy diet comprising of a variety of fruits, vegetables, legumes, nuts, and seeds is still the best source of antioxidants.

Comparing Lifetime Income Options

The greatest fear of the majority of retirees is longevity threat. Now you can buy insurance to protect yourself from the risk of longevity: the danger of your cash being lost. Just as you cover your own home, vehicle, education, etc. for accidents, insurance companies are now providing retirement benefits.

211

Therefore, it's the best form of insurance because your spouse and profit can remain protected even if you fail (die early). Like all insurance companies, you will buy a policy best suited to your needs and circumstances. By comparison to health and life insurance, longevity insurance isn't dependent on your health because you don't live too long, and you don't die too early.

Your pension coverage seems more like an inheritance than insurance. You actually invest any or all of your pension money with an insurance company, and they will then give you an annual living income if you want to cover your spouse. The volume of assured annual income depends on how much money you pay and whether you want single or joint insurance. Let's see how it works.

Suppose you are 55 years old and have started thinking about retirement at the age of 65. During your working years you have been saving money and imagine that you have accrued $300,000 in retirement (this could be in a401(k),403(b), or in an account that does not qualify like insurance, such as shares, bonds, bank cds, leases, real estate, etc.). Let's just assume that in 10 years, you want to make sure that you have at least $50,000 per year when you retire, and this figure is guaranteed over your life. How can you handle this lifetime guaranteed income now ready in 10 years? First, we have to see how much you get from other sources. Let us make this easy by saying that social security is your only other source of income.

You can predict your social security benefits if you go to the website of the Social Security Administration (www.ssa.gov) and make certain assumptions. Let us just assume that and note that in ten years, you plan to retire, and your social security benefits will be $25,803. The job is to see how much the insurance company needs to buy an annuity now, which will ensure the remaining $24,197 when you retire in the next ten years. You want to search on the market for the right investment, and it is usually done by employing the financial advisor's services. Let us assume you consider a fixed index-linked annuity that promises a minimum annual rise in your money if you actually make it income (yes, there are annuities from premium insurance companies that are going to do that).

213

Do believe that you will be compensated by the insurance firm with a bonus of 10% of the money you invest with it-i.e. if you give it $100,000, you will be credited with $110,000 if you earn a lifetime profit later on. Yes, if you shop, these incentives are available.

When you are 65 years of age, you are guaranteed a lifetime annual revenue equivalent to 5.5 percent of your balance, if you were' lock-in' at the age of 65. How much of your 300,000 dollars will it cost to get a guaranteed lifetime income of $24,197, so that you'll still have at least $50,000 for the rest of your life? Since in ten years you'll need 24,197 dollars and we know it is 5.5% of the account value of your pension, we will divide it by 24,197 by 5.5%. The value is $439,945. But for another decade, you won't need this, so we have to determine how much you need to give now to the insurance company. This is where mathematics is difficult and why you need assistance. If your insurance company spent $203,314 today and you were rewarded with a 10 percent bonus and promised the company would expand by at least seven percent annually in the next decade, you would have the $439,945 required if you retired ten years later.

Through buying an insurance policy, you successfully protected your longevity risk. But what if you don't turn 65 or die sooner than you estimated by the insurance company?

Good news and bad news are there! The bad news is that your cash issues are over. The good news is that if you choose a shared life choice, your partner will maintain the income for the rest of his or her life. If you are not married or have not chosen the marriage option, your beneficiary receives the remaining value of your account. The remaining balance value is based on the amount of money you have received, if any, plus the annuity benefit. The earnings are paid based on the market index, with which it is correlated, but you never engage in market losses; however, according to the market index, you are involved in market gains. Therefore, you're guaranteed a minimum rate of return by the insurance company even if the economy loses the cash in the annuity every year. You can't lose in other words, but you can do very well.

And the longevity risk is protected. You simply can't survive your guaranteed income because your insurance company has to pay you before you die, and the social security agency is obligated to pay for the rest of your life. Additionally, when you die too early, you won't lose your annuity income, because your spouse or beneficiaries will die. The world's best! However, if your situation changes (you can win the lottery or get an inheritance), you can continue, stop and store the income, and you will not pay income tax on profits until ten years after you begin withdrawing it. What if in five years you need income? You that start after one year as long as you are 591/2 years old or older, but the sum will be lower than when you wait ten years to go. Will you start at the end of the 10th year? No, you're in charge

When did insurance companies begin to offer such an annuity? Everything's because of the baby boomers. As you know, between 1946 and 1964, 78 million people were born. The population growth began to grow to 62 in 2008, and for the next 18 years, one boomer will turn 62 every 7.5 seconds. So wonder what the greatest thing about them is? Yeah, because they don't have a lifetime pension-like their parents and grandparents did. We turn to the insurance industry to guarantee their living income is too long and to insist that they do not give away their money if they die too soon. The insurance industry has responded.

Is this policy fair to policyholders? We offer protection against a loss like all insurance policies, and in this case, those who die too early don't get a deal as good as those who live too long. But because your number one concern is that your money will survive and you will not be upset that you leave money on the table until you progress to a position where the money is not important, you protected the risk at a fair price. Insurance companies do what they do best: bring the risk together across a large group to ensure that they pay if the worst happens. In this scenario, the worst thing is to live too long for your retirement money. If your mortality risk worries you, contact your financial advisor today and discuss this new type of insurance with him/her. When choosing a rent with a guaranteed lifetime income gain, keep in mind the following:

217

Compare carefully how much money is needed in similar exercises. Get your financial advisor's support!

Compare the rider's costs: they vary between 0 and 0.4 percent annually.

How often do the variables of income change? Every year, every five years, every ten years, etc.

Spousal continuity arrangements and inflation coverage are also in effect.

What are the "step-up" income features offered? As you step up, does the age-related income variable also increase?

How long can you keep your income balance guaranteed?

What is the insurance company's rating?

CHAPTER EIGHT

Can We Live to 150 Years Old?

I hope we, as human beings, will live to the age of 150... Yes, we live in a world full of cynicism and materialism. Those of us who transcend the belief system that culture pressures us and actually interacts with its own internal powers will have the strongest longevity chance. The first step in success is that you believe it can happen. Your belief system's power goes beyond written words. This makes underdogs win overall odds. It is the backbone of most wonders. It might indeed be your first waking to a new journey of a safe and happy life.

I know that many people rely on the information they receive from doctors or what they listen to on TV or in casual conversations. In my quest to find the best foods ever, I researched anti-aging and longevity. I have encountered a lot of key ideas and lifestyle principles that I believe would stack your survival chances if integrated into your life.

For example, I believe that the belief system has a genetic effect on us. It's only important to me. There is an explanation of why your heart rate increases or your hair rise on your legs as you think about things. The same applies to the sensation you get when certain songs come on the radio. The link between your mind and your soul is actually your contact with each cell in your body. You have the power to control your genes by watching what you think and eat. We've always heard you're what you're eating. Do you know what you think? You heard what you think? I think it's just as important because it regulates your stress levels and keeps you safe. Let us look at a rapid action plan that we could start today to make a successful path towards 150 years of age.

I know you've previously heard this, but you must find a way to add additional fruit and vegetables to your diet. Even the current pyramid has raised average intake by 9 to 12 portions per day. This is almost unlikely for most people, so you have to do anything you can to come close to it, even when that means that you can take supplements of fruit and vegetables in capsule or powder. It's a step in the right direction. We also have to stop putting into our bodies toxins. Remove hydrogenated oils, high-fruit corn syrups, pesticides and herbicides, food-sustaining chemicals, dirty water, and dirty air. Dirty air can be hard because so many variables are present. Don't leave all winter shut your doors. Open the windows for at least 15 minutes a day. Plants are another good suggestion. Plants absorb and oxygenate carbon dioxide in your house. Bamboo, Chinese evergreens, Aloe Vera, and spider plants are some healthy oxygenating plants.

We must also combat all the free radicals produced with some healthy antioxidants in our bodies. These are best extracted from fruits filled with 1000 other substances that function together to sustain our immune system and cells. Classic seed extract, Vitamin A, C and E, tomato lycopene, CoQ10, Lipoic acid, L-Carina, and various colorful fruit are also available. Daily exercise is another big help for your body. Strength training is considered in particular to increase human growth hormones that are noted for their anti-aging properties. Most people go to anti-aging clinics, which is a step in the right direction, but strength training will provide some of the same advantages. Sleep is another generator of human growth hormones. Sleep is extremely important, and studies have shown a 60 percent higher mortality rate for people who sleep less than 5 hours or more than 10 hours.

In particular, there are some foods I have read that appear to receive a lot of anti-aging attention. Resveratrol is a well-known anti-aging agent in the skin of vine, grape-seed, peanuts, mulberries, and raspberries except that the majority equates it with red wine. Nevertheless, in my opinion, an excess of red wine decreases the effect due to the impact of the added alcohol on the liver. Coconut oil, which most people unfortunately say is wrong for them, is indeed an excellent commodity. It's good on the body, and it's the only oil that I'm cooking with, and recent studies have seen its anti-aging properties. Omega 3's have always been significantly ovated on the anti-aging front since the Japanese people who consume so much of it have a much longer life than the western world. It is flax seed, hemp seed, avocados, olives, nuts, and Krill oil that I get Omega 3.

Some other items of general interest in the longevity arena are too little to feed. This can be challenging for athletes, in particular, who need fuel carbs. Nevertheless, feeding was mildly shown to help us live longer, if possible, during training periods or for one day here or there. In Russia, tests were done on chickens that lived three times longer than other chickens, fed a small diet rich in organic raw foods. We should also retain as much as possible an alkaline skin. Cancer can not live in an alkaline atmosphere so that eating alkaline food, consuming alkaline water, and managing pressure at the very least keeps you alkaline and helps your body preserve minerals, rather than increasing your alkalinity. Deep breathing is also a good practice because it alleviates the pressure that's a killer. We can all reduce stress, and whatever you do will increase your lifespan. I know it can seem like a full-time business trying to eat healthily, exercise properly, living in a place with great weather, drinking the best water ever, being among the best people to raise their spirits, incorporating organic superfoods and nutrients that are especially useful for you based on your gene profile. But it can also be a way of life and not a full-time job. It's often said that the average of 5 people you hang around will be your net worth. I would suggest that your wellbeing would represent the five people you most often hang around. I know that some people don't seem to control the people they have around them right now. We are trapped in jobs or relationships for whatever reason. It can, however, be a target you set for a life you build, which is safe for you and the people around you. You'll draw healthier people to your life. Many people know these things deep inside. You may not know about specific foods you can consume, but you know when the atmosphere is unhealthy. The key factor is the health of the colon. One likes to talk about it, but it's basically a dangerous region of our body, and the wellbeing is compromised when it doesn't function properly. You need to get fiber into your skin and think about washing. Get a naturopathic doctor who is passionate about health, if possible, in your city. They are worth the expense of the pocket because it's not everything about insurance or the procedure with them. You pay now, or you pay later. In the digestive system and colon, approximately 90 percent of diseases begin.

I assume that you will lighten a spark plug in your lifetime engine by adopting certain of these ideas. It is true that on this planet there are people who have lived very long lives. By putting good food in your skin, you strengthen your genes. Don't get into believing that your genes are lost. Your genes determine just 25 percent or less of your destiny, and your behavior does not affect only the other 75 percent but also causes any "evil" genes you believe you have. The gene is the loaded gun. The catalyst is your lifestyle. You can only live longer than you "say" and do not pull the trigger.

This can be taken to any level you want.

Level A–Xtreme Health (TM) Follow all the advice in this chapter during the next few months, Level B–even better than most people eat more fruits and vegetables, exercise every day, believe that you can live a long life and feel healthy and solid, even when you are over 100 Level Cage–one step further than what you do now stop taking bad foods. Eat organic foods at least one day a week and enjoy the wonderful things the world has brought us.

225

Why Protein Promotes Longevity

Aging, we all want to live long, healthy lives, avoiding the illnesses and diseases that the elderly seem to suffer. The photos of the elderly bent over, limping, walking, and wheelchair are depressing, especially if the person is very much in love with you. But what we can do is just part of getting old. They don't regulate the aging process, right? That's not entirely true, however. We monitor the quality of life that we experience as we get older. And a higher quality of life also means a longer lifespan.

Aging, what's the whole thing? When we grow older, our bodies tend to wear out. The human body is like a car. It has a large number of moving parts that operate together. And as we all know, there's no old car running like a new car. The same goes for the human body. The moving parts of the body include the brain, liver kidneys, and many others. As the body grows older, it becomes vulnerable to harmful radicals. Free radicals continue to weaken and erode our bodies, rendering them more susceptible to disease and disease.

Free radicals can best be combated by eating healthy. The cornerstone of a healthy, disease-free way of life is quality organic food. How we eat in meat and fluids makes a big difference in how happy we are in our later years.

The old saying, "You are what you eat" is very true. A study shows that American centenarians (100 years of age or older) eat 2.5 times more vegetables than seniors under 99 years of age. About five times as many vegetables as 40 years of age. It has also been confirmed that people who eat a lot of fresh organic food do not smoke or drink excess alcohol have higher levels of antioxidants in their bodies, and they live longer. How you eat and stop eating plays an important role in deciding the value and sustainability of your health.

Eating healthy organic foods is good, but we should discuss another equally important aspect of healthy living and supplements. There is convincing evidence that a mixture of L-

Carnitine and Alpha-Lipoic Acid antioxidant has a revitalizing effect on an individual's energy level. It is healthy and has no side effects. Nonetheless, people with diabetes or risk for seizure should avoid these two supplements. Yet Vitamin C, Resveratrol, or Magnesium are not to be avoided. Vitamin C stimulates and reduces inflammation in the immune system. Resveratrol activates the human anti-aging gene (SIRT-1 gene). Magnesium helps strengthen the length of our chromosome protective tips. The three are longevity-friendly and safe to eat. Excessive amounts of vitamin C may be responsible for diarrhea. What is excessive depends on the individual, so take this into account. For example, if you have diarrhea with three caps, take two and enjoy the added bonus of daily bowel movements.

You can be disease-free, physically mature, and it means nothing unless the brain is working properly. Your amygdala is your body's mission control. Do not forget, and I repeat how important it is to maintain a healthy brain. If it doesn't work correctly, it can cause many problems. The brain controls every body function, keeping it alive at all costs. You could spend your older years in a nursing home if you don't.

Let's look at some of the issues we face to keep our brain cells from weakening. This is a subject I am very familiar with. My mom had irreversible brain damage caused by a stroke. I cared for her at home and gradually watched her life quality slip away. It was hard to see that I knew nothing could be done to stop her regression. I promised, in the memory of my mother, to help me avoid a similar situation as much as I could.

We've all heard the phrase, senior moments, what does it mean? When we reach our later years, our brains don't function when well as we did when we were younger, like some of our other organs. We misplace things, forget about the names of people we have known, and sometimes walk into a room to wonder, "What did I come in here for?" By a supplement called Phosphatidyl-Serine (PS), we can reduce or even remove senior moments. This contains the amino acid serine and essential fatty acids present in almost every cell membrane. Our cells had an abundance of PS during our younger years,

229

everything we wanted. But, as we get older, our PS rates decrease. PS is important because it activates memory, attention, vocabulary, and learning capabilities in the brain area. PS can also reduce dementia symptoms, anxiety, Alzheimer's disease, and the harmful effects of stress. As of this writing, Alzheimer's disease is not healed, but PS helps alleviate certain symptoms.

PS has a twin called Phosphatidyl-Choline (PC), a brain boost supplement that gives choline to the skin. PC is a major component of lecithin that has proven to be an important addition to improved memory. Of example, the combined use of PC and PS will greatly improve the memory capacity.

Exercise in senior citizens has long been associated with connective brain function. But don't wait for you to begin a workout program until you are a senior citizen. Do it now because exercise improves the brain and all parts of the body's blood circulation. Go for a stroll if you have limited mobility. If you haven't worked in a while, start slowly, then gradually increase your pace. When you walk, try to walk briskly five days a week for 30 minutes.

When we age, we lose muscle mass regularly. This is often an indirect cause of the many interactions of senior citizens. A senior can preserve, even increase, dietary muscle mass, supplementary, and weight exercise. Using protein is certainly a good idea if you want to include weight training in your routine. Protein not only increases muscle mass but also comprises much of our inner tissue. Whey Protein should be a good choice of your protein supplement.

Whey Protein Promotes Longevity Research has found that our senior population is upset. It seems that 45% of our seniors in the general population and 85% to 100% of our elderly in healthcare facilities are malnourished. This is due to poor appetite caused by drug side effects and a variety of other serious but preventable conditions, including patient abuse and neglect.

The factor that contributes is inadequate absorption of a high-quality protein, leading to a decrease in muscle weight, decreased strength, reduced bone mass, delayed surgical regeneration, decreased immunity, and various other body disorders. Combining such issues would inevitably result in the ultimate senior issue, fragility. These issues may be avoided by whey protein. Whey is a high-quality protein supplement highly recommended for the elderly. The origin of BCAA is rich in branch-chain amino acids to promote protein synthesis and prevent the breakdown of protein. But Whey provides calorie reducing benefits. So how does it translate into longevity? The life expectancy today is 78.7 years. When you begin a Whey plan in the middle of your life, you can expect 9.5 years to increase your lifespan.

Research has proven that Whey is superior to other protein supplements in the suppression of cancer cell growth. More studies have shown that the tumor prevention abilities of Whey have been accompanied by its increased levels of glutathione accompanied by the element Lactoferrin, which inhibits tumor formation intensively.

232

Aging Is a Treatable Disease

Live healthily–look awesome–live longer. You can and will do it today to significantly improve your health, appearance, and longevity. You can control 70% of the factors that affect your survival, but just 30% are biologically determined by genetic regulation at a late stage of your life. The keys are early detection and early treatment.

Our understanding of the aging process advances rapidly. Many scientists believe that the first eternal human can be today.

Life expectancy in 1786 was 24 years. Good diets and some medical advances helped it double to 48 years in the next 100 years.

Today, the life expectancy of modern medicine has increased to over 76 years. Future medicine hopes to lift it to over 100 years of our lives.

233

"Over half of baby boomers in America today are in excellent health for their 100th birthday and beyond," "we look at the baby boomers ' life and the generation of post-baby boomers from 120 to 150 years old." The key to living healthy, Look marvelous, is to slow down aging illnesses, so they are very late in life.

The causes of aging are finally understood. You should take action today to take advantage of recent medical developments. Dr. Rudman performed a number of experiments on elderly people to prevent and reverse the effects of aging. The cause of aging Almost every earth's life flowers with young people before they regenerate and pass on genes to the next generation. "It is not inevitable that the body will eventually become aged," he said. "The flowers waved and died, and we humans started to age. Of course, we continue to age while we're still in our twenties.

We mature, although the effects of our metabolism, i.e., our' balls,' accumulate more rapidly from the oxidation process that

234

produces energy in our cells than our endocrine system. This is because most healing hormones in our young bodies begin to decline as we age. Some of these more essential hormones dropped by about 10 to 30 percent in our 30s. Once we hit the next decades, the losses are very dramatic. Most of our hormones have fallen by more than 50%, and some have dropped to almost zero as we hit our 70s. And we're aging. And we age. So we age. Weaken our bones and muscles, slow down our reaction time, lose our strength, all of which combine in order to make us more unintentionally vulnerable. The immune system weakens and makes us more vulnerable to diseases. And we are dying. And we are dying.

Another cause of aging has been shown by Dr. Hayflick's death clock. He showed that we have an integrated deadline of about 120 years if we do not have diseases or injuries. This date of death is when our cells have split many times. Our cells divide to produce new cells to replace the old cells that were destroyed with metabolic debris, free radicals, toxins, and other forms of wear and tear. The cells divide, and the chromosomes separate to provide chromosomes to the new cells. As

235

chromosomes divide, they lose part of their telomeres, which are divided by the genes that carry chromosomes. Following a number of breaks, the telomeres become weary and too small to maintain a chromosome, so that the cell dies and can not replace itself.

Telomers can be seen at the ends of the shoelaces as plastic lines. Telomeres hold intact the basic DNA code in order not to duplicate it as the molecules reproduce over time.

Nevertheless, experiments over recent years have shown that the Hayflick cap can be extended by using an enzyme that can re-widen "organizing genes" at the end of chromosomes (telomeres). The enzyme is believed to be telomerase.

Telomerase studies have shown in human laboratory cells that telomerase can immortalize human cells. Doctors and scientists who engage in these treatments agree that death is not inevitable.

Therefore, telomerase is an enzyme (a catalytic protein), which prevents or reverses the telomere shortening cycle. When we are embryos in the womb, the body produces telomerase to help the embryo grow very quickly. Our bodies, however, do not, unfortunately, contain telomerase after birth, except for the production of sperm.

In order to extend life for men, we must do two things. Next, oxidants and contaminants must be eliminated from food, and the atmosphere and a nutrient or therapeutic mechanism are sought for the development and maintenance of the lengths of our cells ' telomeres.

Promising anti-aging research Many programs are currently underway to deal with our aging problems. One is from a group of South Korean scientists. You say that you arc making a newly synthesized molecule, CGK733, that can make cells younger.

"We avoided dividing cells, and in the end, we saw that the process was interrupted by the CGK733," Professor Kim Tae-

Kok said. In less than ten years, Kim hopes that CGK733-enhanced drugs that keep cells younger than average will be sold. "It is also probable that the synthetic compound will revitalize aging by revitalizing the already lethargic cells.

Wistar Institute scientists have identified a key objective of an adaptive protein that regulates the aging process. Work offers fundamental knowledge of critical aging mechanisms leading to new anti-aging and cancer therapies.

Aging threatens, paralyzes, and destroys our strength and ability to enjoy life. Tens of millions die each year from conditions associated with age. Very few people know that decisions on diet and lifestyle, medicines and nutraceuticals will delay degenerative aging.

Very few are aware of the many serious scientific attempts to understand and intervene with the aging process one day to reverse its effects.

The goal should be to live a healthy life and long enough to take advantage of all current medical advancements and developments.

Our wellbeing is dependent on our past and presents genes, diets, and behaviors. You can actually improve your current and future health by identification and taking herbal products, vitamins, and other nutrients and therapies tailored to your particular health needs. The plan acknowledges the significance of three key themes: medicine's future in person-friendly medicine: key aging is a treatable disease.

You will read about the latest anti-aging knowledge and develop your own longevity plan. The key to a longer life is that emerging tools are recognized and used to address health challenges as quickly as possible. Time is important, really.

Lifetime Wellness System

We enter a new age of fitness and nutrition. Money isn't the most important thing we want to do anymore. We see how people have lost their careers and jobs in their lives and continue to survive. Families are together to support each other. Total strangers meet each other. In this new era of growth, health, and inner harmony are emerging. The placement of happiness and health is high on the priority list. Without these resources, money does not mean much, and it does not help either.

For centuries people believed in and relied entirely on the health and wellbeing of their medical profession. It is a thing of the past to take whatever drugs the doctor prescribed and to do anything the doctor ordered without a doubt. Social empowerment is developing today. People ask questions, refuse to take prescription medicines blindly without understanding the side effects, and inquire for alternative approaches. People take responsibility for their own health, wellbeing, and wellbeing. In so doing, we have often found that we do well without all the medications and side effects. We are looking for alternatives to nature. It is important to rip our bodies of years of accumulated toxins held in our bodies due to multiple prescription medications, poor eating habits, sleeplessness, and unnecessary stress, and a constant worry to ensure a longer life.

The DIET concept has a new meaning, and it is no longer DIE-AT-IT. Diet now means changing your mindset and attitude to an entire lifestyle that requires nourishing the body and making it easier to digest. We discover that a healthy weight can be reached by eating healthier foods. Foods without chemical additives, artificial flavors, or colors, and no chemicals make losing weight easier because your body gets the nutrients it needs and feels full and satisfied. Therefore there is no need to binge.

We show you our Anti Aging Lifetime Wellness Program to learn to calm your mind, to relax completely from the inside without drugs or alcohol. Stress causes sickness, pain, anxiety, and many other issues in nutrition.

Why are cancer and diabetes so prevalent? What are the causes of these diseases? Why isn't there any cure? This is a treatment for these and many other illnesses that have ravaged our world

241

like a relentless and persistent epidemic. The solution is clear. It is referred to as natural life. I said simple, not easy. I said, simply. This means prioritizing your health and wellbeing if you want to achieve longevity. This includes making a conscious effort to purchase products that do not harm us in or on our bodies. Such items are harder to find and often cost more, so they are moved to the shelf to something more affordable. Since only a small percentage of the population has become aware that many products that are currently easily available are not healthy, they cost more. This small percentage of the population has already assigned #1 priority to their wellbeing. Price also depends on supply and demand. If the populace requested a higher percentage of healthy goods, the number of healthy products would be greater and more economical. We allowed what is available and cheap to determine how we live.

When baby boomers achieve adulthood, the climate shifts tremendously. One by each baby boomer reaffirm his priorities and reassess his choices in order to ensure a happy, energetic life that includes living in his own home for healthy and independent years because he is healthy and good enough to do so. Rather than focusing on living in a nursing home or spending their last few years in depression and loneliness, it is clear that it makes much more sense to change the quality of life NOW to have a better feeling. Our Anti Aging Lifetime Wellness Program offers a number of different alternative medicine and wellness programs, from the treatment of lamps, a calming wall of water, enhanced memory and concentration, visual enhancement, and reinforced muscle eyes through to the Rejuvenator Machine.

You would be safer if you stopped buying three cheap, synthetic cloths imported from a country that probably still produces formal or another chemical and purchased one piece of natural material. Your skin might breathe. When you eat healthier food, you will find that you don't feel that you have to eat so much. The way the human body interprets and uses the food and beverage provides influences the capacity of the body to metabolize and regenerate cells. The human body does not consider all foods and diet drinks with artificial ingredients, chemicals, and chemical additives as the nutrition it requires

243

and does not, therefore, meet the requirements, so that you eat and drink, and therefore gain weight. Because your digestive system is now bloated with toxins, it takes all your strength to plug your body into the sofa and eat the mess. But watch pointless TV, you have no energy left for anything.

Let's analyze this...

1. By buying cheap, organic clothing that covers your skin 24 hours a day, you have saved some money. You experience itches or rashes, prompting you to look for a cure, whether it is a visit to a doctor like a dermatologist or an otherwise topical cream and wonder... What's wrong?

2. By buying cheap food filled with pesticides, additives, hormones, and artificial ingredients, you saved money. You had to eat much more to the full, so it cost more money. You gain weight, and you don't have strength, you feel awful. You're going to your doctor and saying... What's wrong?

3. You are taking prescription drugs, and now you feel even worse. You have pain, you can't sleep, and you feel depressed.

Further visits by doctors, tests, a lot of screening, MRI, CAT Scan, PET Scan, etc. All this costs money, money, and time. When you ask... What is wrong, there are no reasons or answers?

4. You wash your hair with a mixture of artificial coloring, additives, and fragrances. Your hair is unable to stand against such torture, so it gets brittle, breaks off and looks awful. You buy special conditioners and shampoos filled with artificial dyes to save your skin desperately. It does not work. It does not work. You are forced to wear your hair far shorter than you want, but there is no choice at this point. You're going to the beauty store and wondering... What's wrong?

5. You take a shower with soap filled with additives, softeners, fake teeth, and artificial colors at least once a day, and add body lotions that are also poisonous. Regular shower further endangers your wellbeing by aggravating hair/body lotion poisoning because this toxic process is repeated. The more chemicals you use, wear, or add to your skin, the more toxins you build up. Your sweat Smells Bad as your cells breathe and

try to survive ongoing abuse. When you didn't eat toxins, wear artificial garments, and cover your skin with chemical additives, your body wouldn't sweat, and more than once, you could wear an outfit until you were cleaned.

It occurs to me that all these problems are directly linked to an increasing global health crisis. This can be corrected only in one way. Every person has to take personal responsibility for his own health and wellness, which means starting to make changes right now.

Start reading and learning what you eat, read the labels, and purchase food and other items without additives. Drink filtered water to flush your body's toxins. Begin an ongoing training program. Walking isn't necessary. If walking succeeded, every woman in the mall looked great, and you didn't. Take care of your life.

CHAPTER NINE

What Is Holistic Health?

People of all ages are concerned with their health, their feelings, their looks, the prevention of diseases, and the quality of life. The majority of societies have recently been brainwashed to agree in excessive exercise, less fat, medications, , Botox injections as the solution to safety, fertility, longevity, and fat loss.

How would you obtain perfect wellbeing without gimmicks and artificial fixes, of course? Winning fitness, strength, resilience, and fat loss are multidimensional wellness approaches that include all facets of wellbeing, including body, mind, emotion, atmosphere, culture, and spiritual wellbeing. Holistic nutrition is a lifestyle that allows you to take an active interest in the monitoring and responsibility of different things in your life, including

• the Sensitive exercise program • Complementary medication • Wholistic diet, organic food • Emotional and mental

wellbeing • Optimal digestion — Periodic detoxification •
Positive thought and mental wellbeing. This includes peace of
mind, joy, and full wellbeing at all stages-physically,
psychologically, socially, mentally, and spiritually. It is an
evolution, balance, and integration. You consist of mind, spirit,
and body. If one of these areas has a problem, it will affect the
others.

The application of holistic health principles can minimize
many symptoms of health, including chronic stress,
degenerative diseases, lifestyle disorders, and hormonal
imbalances, high cholesterol, obesity, glandular weakness, gut
disorder, and a decreased functioning immune system.

The individual with a bronzed tan does not show holistic health,
a chiseled six-pack abdominal eating 800 calories a day. It's not
also the person jogging 25 miles a week, the latest celebrity
diet, or the person who has undergone one artificial chirurgy
after another.

The reality is that no exercise or cosmetic operation will shape
your physical condition without paying attention to your
lifestyle, emotions, and safe diet. Most diets make you crash.

They work against your natural biochemistry and plan to store your body fat.

Diets and loss of weight lead to endangered metabolism.

People who maintain their natural weight typically have a good connection to food and see it as nutrition. We enjoy food and cooking without feeling guilty, nervous, or distracted.

The American population has been misinformed about the weight loss, basic science, and a healthy lifestyle.

Self-acceptance is a key component of wellness. Most conclude that at the age of 40, their intellect, their vision, their ears, their libido, their joints, and their bodies are weakening and degenerate. Worse, society has become dependent on the most basic human functions through pharmaceuticals, stimulants, and processed food.

Many use drug addictions, sugar, and other chemical stimulants. Those make your power deplete, damage your health, and make you more depleted. Both addictions are triggered by internal emotional conflict.

With regard to four factors, 90 percent of all illnesses could be avoided: stress control, sunshine, nutrition, and exercise.

249

Sadly, medical schools will teach potential doctors little, if any, on food, fitness, or disease prevention. Alternatively, physicians were told how to administer dangerous substances, making physicians the third leading cause of death. The Rx drug serves as a band-help. This worsens or reappears, in another manner after a period of time. Every patent medicine has a list of side effects that often complicate problems. Further medications are ultimately needed to deal with them, leading to the destruction of biochemistry and eventual death.

The whole person and their lifestyle are concerned with holistic health. This focuses on prevention, nutrition, wellbeing, and longevity. You are an active participant in your life's healing process or a passive beneficiary.

Do what most Americans are doing (avoid exercise, eat a large share of their fast food, alcohol and Junk food diets, eat white fours and white sugar, skip medication and instead take prescribed drugs that prematurely age the liver, pancreas, kidney and other organs).

VITALITY, HEALTH WING, FAT LOSS, and LONGEVITY

Water: Drink plenty of water. Each metabolism in your body needs to be completed with water. Do you try to lose body fat, relieve constipation, headaches, or low back pain? Drink more water. Drink more water. The equation for you is to take your body weight and multiply by seven, and this will help you to drink the number of ounces of water every day. To maximize absorption and cellular hydration, add a pinch of Celtic sea salt. Adding lemon to your water prevents kidney stone production, creates an alkaline environment, and nourishes your liver. Moderate exercise: The body Should keep healthy, strong, and young every day. The intensity and frequency of your workout plan depending on your fitness and health overall. Unfortunately, most people tend to under-exercise or over-exercise.

Excessive cardiovascular exercise has a huge effect on the hormone levels of a woman. You can actually overdo cardiovascular exercise to deplete the sex hormones. This often affects women more rapidly than men and raises their effects with a woman reaching her 40s and entering menopause. A woman's metabolism from years of aerobic activity is continually restored and slowed down with adverse hormonal consequences. Most people believe that cardiovascular exercise is the perfect workout, as they then feel refreshed and energized. This is only because the surreal medications were overstimulated, and ample adrenaline and cortisol were secreted.

Several studies have shown that aerobic exercise does not promote muscle growth. Yes, cardiovascular exercise effectively inhibits muscle growth and can also reduce muscle mass, rendering it ineffective.

I'm not alone against aerobics. Three of the top medical and physical health experts all recommend against cardiovascular exercise, as it creates high levels of stress on the skin, depletes — cardiovascular exercise.

The average woman performs endless hours of exercise/aerobics, does not have endurance exercises; hunger focuses on the numbers and wonders why her body does not improve for all its effort and time.

My winning strategy for muscle building and reducing your fat shops means lifting weights daily for 45-50 minutes, at least two or three days a week, with a full-body training program.

Nutrition: eat foods entirely, unprocessed, preferably organic. Commercially farmed animals are flooded with hormones, antibiotics, and other drugs that stimulate growth. Organic foods not only provide nutrients with higher densities required for the detoxification of the skin.

Take the time to cook your own meals instead of depending on fast food. You are what you eat. You are what you eat. Make sure you eat a lean, quality protein source breakfast every day. Think PVFC (veggie, protein, carbohydrate, healthy fat) while preparing meals.

Your body needs high-nutritional foods in comparison to fast foods or junk foods that are VOIDs without nutritional value. Your body's nutrients actually cost you to absorb and process fast food. If you do not provide the food you need to function properly, it will degenerate and cause a host of health issues. DO NOT underestimate the good food quality. Food is medicine. You are what you eat. You are what you eat.

Eliminating toxins: toxins from food additives, preservatives, dry cleaners, pesticides, and contaminants are exposed to us. the average American has 116 chemical substances in his skin. Reduce meat, sugar, milk, caffeine, and alcohol consumption. Eliminate all derivatives containing high-fructose maize syrup and/or partially hydrogenated trans fats absolutely.

What you need to know is this - if you want to alter the shape of your body, your liver has to remove all the toxins brought into your body by your food. In your fat cells, toxins are contained. It is hard to lose body fat when you are stressed, and your liver is congested.

Sleep: Sleep can be very well the' youth pool.' Research by the National Health Institute indicates that from 10 p.m. And 2 a.m. And at 2 a.m. The physical regeneration of your body takes place between 2 a.m. hours. And at 6 a.m. And at 6 a.m. Regeneration occurs mentally and emotionally. The earlier you will live until 10:30 p.m. And as the body and mind will relax and heal by 6:00 a.m.

When you stay continuously until 10:30 p.m., your growth and repair hormones (they will below) are likely to have imbalances with your stress hormones (they will be high). Pressure management: Stress is like dark chocolate–a little's all right, but much's going to kill you. Stress, weight gain, and obesity have been linked with almost all major diseases. When you are stressed out, the stress hormone secreted by the adrenal glands is the steady influx of cortisol in your body. It causes

254

the body's mechanisms to fail slowly and leads to premature aging, excess belly fat, degeneration, and finally, diseases. The remainder may take the form of relaxation for 20 minutes, a moist soothing bath with Epsom salts and lavender, revived yoga, or religious or uplifting learning. Take a look at your relationships, check your accounts, look at your daily schedule, and commit to removing anything that does not improve your life. Manage your' to - do' list, set boundaries, volunteers, pets, and other stressful busters, listen to classical music, spend time on nature or the sea.

Respiration: Deep breathing is the source of all your body's energy. This releases endorphins that generate joy. Deep breathing revitalizes every cell in your body and stimulates them. Without enough oxygen, cells start to die, and energy is not created enough. Practice deep, full breathing into your belly every day for 5 minutes of solitude. One example is inhaling four counts, holding four counts, exhaling eight counts, and holding four counts. You will note an enormous difference in energy, mood, and clarity.

Spiritual connection: You are essential for balance and harmony in your desire to communicate at a soul level. The way you choose your spiritual connection can include: being surrounded by similar religious people, prayer, the reading of something sacred, reflection, and /or isolation in nature.

A balanced digestive system: you can consume the best food on the planet, but you will not ingest, assimilate, metabolize, or remove food molecules correctly if your digestive system does not work properly. Most illnesses and diseases are caused by a malfunctioning digestive system. 70% of your immune system is in the digestive tract.

Tips for digestion improvement:

1. Drink two glasses of water 15 minutes before every meal with a lemon juice. Taking hydrochloric acid levels in the stomach during a meal dilutes and weakens digestion.

2. Chew your food until it has been liquefied.

3. Take digestive enzymes and HCl into consideration.

4. Don't eat under pressure! Do not watch the news, chat noisy, hear loud music, eat quickly, or read stressful details while cooking.

Provide objectives: Set short, mid-term, and long-term goals to be realistic and achievable. Write them down. Write them down. This means that you have made a major commitment to them and are much more likely to follow your strategy.

Keep a positive view. You can imagine that this is much more relevant. Chronic stress speeds up aging and causes disease. Those who feel happier on average have lower levels of the stress hormone, cortisol, which is linked to high blood pressure and type II diabetes.

Negative mental and emotional stress leads to your health and causes imbalances and diseases. Changing your perspective will affect the neurochemistry of your brain. A good attitude can keep you well into old age, healthy, happy, and alive. A further WINNING FORMULA is to live in thanks to the potentially deadly effects of stress. Make a list of 10 things every day for which you are grateful. These will immediately shift your energy. You're going to feel better and less depressed. Concentrate on positive results and desired behavior. Positive emotional factors are correlated with extended life expectancy.

The Delicacy of pH Balance in the Body

Of all the millions for processes that take place minutes by minutes in your body, the pH rate in your blood and in your cells is one of the most important to keep in optimal balance. The body uses countless amounts of energy to ensure that the pH in your bloodstream and in all other cells is held at its right level. The strength of your pH determines whether or not your body can work the way it should. Your organs make up the "systems" of your body, so they also depend on a proper pH balance. Such systems could include your digestive system (breaks down and absorbs nutrients from the food you eat), your cardiovascular system (correction and circulation), your immune system (fights infection). The proper balance of your pH levels at the cellular level allows the body the ability to bear unnecessary waste and toxins from cells as well. It protects the blood and its ability to transport oxygen to cells and has a large number of other important health roles.

The balance of these pH levels in the appropriate range is one of the biggest "balancing activities" for the body. There is a constant battle in the body to regulate the pH level. The food we eat and the liquids we drink decide whether or not the internal structures are kept in an acidic or alkaline state. The acidic environment breaks down body defenses while an alkaline state contributes to life, nutrition, healing, and longer life. The leeway margin for this pH balance is very low, and the body must maintain the same level to ensure that your processes work the way they should. There is never a time when the body will "drop the ball" and stop doing what is needed to control the pH, particularly at mealtimes. The big problem is that we make it too hard for the body to work in a healthy life-producing pH environment.

You see, when we break down in the digestive tract, all foods that we consume contain a residue called "ash." The residue of "ash" is left over the material after the body uses the fuel from the food we eat. The threat to our pH begins with our chewing and mixing food with saliva in our mouth. The nutrition then passes into our digestive stomach or is literally separated into its components. Then it is passed to our intestines where the nutrients that break down our food are consumed in the digestive process (if all goes well). The foods we eat decide if there is a trace of ACID "dust," or if that is an ALKALINE "ash" that is created in the body.

The big problem is that most of us eat most of our foods that produce acid ash that pushes the pH levels of the body to the acid range-exactly where it NOT belongs. The cellular level of the body is designed to work best if it is in a limited ALKALINE array. The body and cells work with the highest efficiency in this alkaline environment.

In an acid environment, the intestines become a virtual breeding ground for parasites and bacterial infestations that lead to high disease sensitivity. The gut also stays alkaline and creates an environment of equilibrium, harmony, and symbiotic homeostasis in the right alkaline state. It simply means that the engine firs on all cylinders without having to work harder than expected. You want to create a toxic, acidic, anaerobic, and parasite-infested intestinal environment that causes disease? Or would you prefer to give your body an oxygen-rich, alkaline, and essential immunity that is capable of fighting infection and illness in the best way possible?

Your choice is yours. The dilemma is that we can not always eat the way we should and drink the right type of water to ensure that the body has the proper pH balance. In fact, how many of us actually eat 3-4 portions of fruit and 5-6 portions of vegetables a day to maintain our pH balance and to produce good health? How many of us drink 8-10 glasses of pure, safe, and alkaline water a day to help our bodies remove our cells ' waste products? Most of us don't come close at all. If these cellular waste products and our toxins and poisons are not removed immediately, they contribute more to an acidic environment in the cells. This has been shown by numerous studies performed over the last 20 years to cause disease, disease, and illness in the body.

Okay, if you are like most Americans, we're not taking the time to do the stuff you need to support us. We usually wait for something in the body to break down and show signs and complications that we can not deal with before we take care of the body. But be inspired, I got great news! It is not as complicated as you might assume to keep your pH at an optimal level. You don't have to stay in the kitchen and eat 16 times a day to get the correct pH level back into the cells. Many drugs have been specifically formulated to restore the pH levels in your blood, cells, organs, and body systems. Such products are great for their ability to restore the pH balance in a simple and simplistic way to its optimum alkalinity. The first comes in a line of puffers, usually called' natural drinks,' which you mix in juice or water, allowing the body to respond to alkalinity instantly. As you probably know, any kind of dietary help does not completely replace the need for a proper diet and cleanse your body, but it takes you a long way to improve health as those changes happen. The goods may also be in the form of an alkaline powder based on fruit, which is good to taste and blends well with juice or water. Nearly immediately, it is absorbed by the body because it is already fluid and needs no lengthy digestive process to break it down, and it works immediately.

Alkalizing drops are the second drug in the arsenal to maintain the pH in the optimum range. This is the easiest way to restore the pH of your body to an optimal level I have ever seen. Men literally carry it in a pants pocket, and because of the very small size of the bottle, women can carry a small bottle or a handbag. It's an exciting advance in a bottle of "portable food." Only a few drops into anything you drink, and you're catapulted into a more functional state in your body. A few important products can be transported with you anywhere you go.

The value of the body for health and longevity cannot be overstated in an alkaline environment. Both of these drugs are useful to protect the body from sickness and disease caused by acid pH in the body.

How Old Are You Really? Biological Age

Individuals have always desired to be "early young," and society today is no different. We want to stop the process of aging.

The rate at which we age can be determined-the so-called biological age, or how old the body really is. Longitude, previously called anti-aging, is the research field extremely popular in the states.

It is something I'm really involved in and see for myself and my clients as a major part of the future.

Your chronological age is just how old you are.

Biological age is really the biological age of the body.

263

Today we will discuss how you can assess your biological age and how you can enhance it.

The list includes a number of longevity factors that shocked me!

First and foremost, people want to be happy. Very easily said than done. Easier said.

Happiness is a mental state. This is a feeling. It is a feeling.

Tell someone with a major objective (such as building a successful company or losing more than three stones)

"What is your goal to do?" They sometimes say something like, "I'll be delighted when I get there" or "satisfied with myself" or say, "I'm proud."

"I'm going to have more energy."

"I'm not afraid to try new things or go out with family."

"I don't want to feel like a food slave" "I don't want to be scared or waver in the mirror."

Everything is all about emotions. All about feelings.

Citizens spend their whole lives looking for feelings! Whether people actually enter this state of "joy" is special for us all (mostly happiness, fulfillment, and love).

Many people I've met AIM with great money for good jobs (or businesses)

264

Everything with the ultimate objective of a good retirement.

I hear someone say, "I'm supposed to do this when I finish work, or I'll... (insert goal)."

The message here, being happy, and having a good retirement is the main purpose of people's lives, will certainly keep your body fit and healthy.

I know that a very wealthy man who had cancer and died just before his retirement was not part of the Master Plan, that he had built his company so that he could sell and retire (as most people do).

He didn't do it and couldn't "cash out."

Most people don't retire because their "project" is chaotic from the very beginning.

Without sounding sad, we recall just one clip.

It's NOT a reproach.

Most men are disabled, and their bodies are ruined!

It keeps them from loving their time off as much. Living life with many restrictions. "Because of the steep hill, I can not go there," or "Because of my back or the knees, I can't do that."

After 40-50 years of hard work–a good pension and a good retirement–this is the last thing anyone needs.

The bodies of the people are like cars.

Firstly, you have new high-kilometer cars that are not well serviced.

On the other side, you have old low-kilometer cars well cared for.

I want you to be like a well-managed old car, with a small milestone when you retire.

I know some people, this walk, I feel and look as if they are 50 or 60 years old!

I know many people who are retired and who feel like being 40 years old, and who can continue to work and work for another 20 years!

All of this depends on how we live our lives; obviously, things like injuries, illnesses, and other bad things can have a negative impact on our lives through our own fault, but we have control over our own health.

What has an effect on our longevity?

Scientists agree that in any way, big or small, these factors affect the lifespan. Muscular size and strength Level of education How healthy you are when you go to see your doctor if necessary The number of friends you can count on and the love you give to in your life Your diet Blood pressure Your strength if you like your job or not Either you smoke or drink alcohol or not and the amount Whether you exercise or not Most of us shorten our life and last but not least

As you might expect, the progression of aging can be delayed and even somewhat reversed.

I would say that with aging, there is nothing wrong; it's unavoidable. We should be proud of this, an opportunity for the younger generation to demonstrate our wisdom.

This chapter shows you how you can safely and appreciate the aging process.

The aging process As you get older, your body slows down and stops functioning as well. Unfortunately, you don't get away from it.

But we can delay our body in years by healthy living and making the right choices day after day!

Only consider how much more can you enjoy your retirement if you feel like you are 40 years old? And the people you love will spend it.

Compare it with how much you will love if you can only walk up a staircase flight without tired legs and breathlessness.

It does not have to be the same or worse your chronological age than your physiological age.

How to slow down the effects of aging The above list obviously helps you, but here are a few more suggestions to beat your time.

That sums up some of the western worlds that most people (facial surgery is an extreme example) take such steps to ensure themselves look much younger rather than healthier and exercise.

Aging contributes to the loss of muscle mass, cognitive function loss, reduced mobility, and strength, and because you know the superficial type of anti-aging measures I have described won't help.

Top tips for naturally slowing aging: enjoy the outdoors—don't spend the entire time behind your screen, or watch TV indoors. There is a lot to do and see outdoors, particularly on a warm day I can't think of anything any better than walking around the park or beach with the kids. Sunlight is also a natural vitamin D source.

Yoga & Meditation-I'd say this is one of the most effective young stay techniques. I started to do this myself, and frankly, it makes me feel great. Yoga and meditation will help you relax and dramatically reduce your stress (connected to aging). It can also allow you to see things much more clearly.

Yoga is also perfect for your endurance, and the more relaxed and agile you are, the lower the risk of pain and disability drops in the future.

Socializing-Loneliness can be a real assassin. Socialize with your friends and family as much as possible. Go out there and do stuff, go to the movies, concerts, engage in an evening class (more relaxing mentally, the better).

Stay Strong & Healthy-You will move constantly, or your body stops. It is absolutely vital to engage in regular exercise. Regular strength training is key.

Losing muscle mass is something you want to stop or at least delay as long as you can, and strength training can help keep your bones healthy and reduce your chances of osteoporosis.

Nutrition I accept that food is medicine; many of the benefits that you get from modern medicine are the right foods.

Nutrition has an effect on biochemistry. Biochemistry affects all at the cellular level.

If you eat well, any medicines should not be required.
It will also demonstrate if you spend the whole of your life eating fresh, whole organic foods and remain active. In the last few days, you will hopefully be lean, mobile, free of diseases, and full of energy.
You should consider eating a diet that contains lots of quality fats and proteins (bodybuilding materials) that helps you maintain your muscle reserves. Protein also increases your body's production of HGH, and HGH (Human Growth Hormone) is the natural' young fountain' of your body.
As you age, this hormone's development slows down considerably, daily force exercise (lifting, pushing, and pulling heavy material), and high-quality protein keeps this hormone produced!

Eat lots of foods rich in antioxidants— antioxidants present in colorful fruits and vegetables help reduce the damage done by free radicals in your body.

Free radicals can accelerate the onset of aging and are unstable electrons (O1) released during metabolism. We destroy the mitochondria and the cell nucleus.

Free radicals bounce like a pinball inside your cells, causing damage to something each time they hit. They are absolutely destructive.

Antioxidants supply the additional O1 molecules to the free radical that must become stable O2 molecules.

Natural foods of good quality are the best way to fight these dangerous free radicals. Natural foods are filled with antioxidants to neutralize free radicals before too much damage is caused.

Lower sugar intake— Excess sugar that you eat can remove essential proteins in the body that can lead to wrinkles and loss of energy — lower sugar intake.

Stop smoking and reduce the consumption of alcohol-Few things age faster than smoking and drinking alcohol daily to quit smoking and to do as much to drink less.

Lower stress rates–This is another major one, and I just said that you age a few things more quickly than cigarettes or alcohol; well, I think stress is one of them.

Stress will kill your mood, power, social interaction, and cause so many health problems.

As I said, I found deep breathing, yoga, and meditation very helpful and a perfect way to fight stress.

People who buy these products don't have to change their lifestyle a bit, that's why they are so famous.

Essentially, if you have put time and effort into your "health & fitness account," you will be able to reap the benefits of our retirement.

If you haven't, you're not going to!

In reality, you can calculate your biological age online with a biological age machine.

When all the points I made above did not require effort or dedication, then everybody would run around in their 90s and later!!

But we don't, unfortunately, die a lot younger than that.

Depending on the figures, UK men have been reported to live on average until 77 or 78 in 2010, while women live on average until 82 or 83 years old.

Do it, of course, and do it correctly.

Let me know what you're thinking about this, post down, I want to know what you're thinking.

CHAPTER TEN

Increased Longevity - What Every Woman Needs to Know Before They Retire

America n women have taken tremendous steps to improve their overall financial outlook and close the income gap with men. Over the last two decades, many women have been educated and self-reliant about their financial future more than their mother ever dreamed of. "Today, for example, third more women graduate from college than men, and 60% of women with a Business Degree receive their husbands." In the last decade, too, the number of women earning 100,000 dollars or more annually quadrupled.

Women have steadily increased their wages and economic strength over the years, but women face many unique challenges when it comes to financial future planning. Women must be mindful of the set of factors that separate them from other countries in America when trying to build on their economic potential and secure their financial future.

Enhanced longevity The disparities in life expectancy between men and women are a distinctive and sometimes ignored trait of America n N women. Females will usually expect to live seven years longer than men on average., people who were born in the United States in 1982 were expected to live 70.8 years. Women born in the same year usually live for 78.1 years. This increased longevity for women poses many obstacles for women in order to build a sound financial strategy. In many cases, as women are expected to survive, they need to prepare for more available income, retirement years for the order to preserve their lifestyle and autonomy.

Yes, all America ns live longer than ever before as a result of developments in health science. As a result, most people enjoy their senior days for up to 20 years or more. Upon query, the majority of pensioners in America saw their number one worry about pensions as the possibility of surviving their pension savings. The effects of inflation and higher taxes make this a

275

real problem for pensioners in America. The increased chances of a long retirement should be an important factor in addressing its retirement plan priorities for current and future women retirees.

Although, over the years, more women have entered America, more often, they continue to play traditional motherly roles in their households, such as raising children and the chief caregiver for the whole family. Women are still the most likely family members to offer career aspirations to elderly parents, children, or spouses with disabilities. In some figures, women, on average, "would lose $550,000 by wages and benefits (including social security) by taking time off from work for family care."

For many women, living longer often means surviving their own primary carers— their husbands. It also raises the risk of seeking the care of a nursing home due to sickness and injury. The majority of women, more than 50 percent (as opposed to 33 percent of men) at age 65, are expected to require care before they die. Although the Medicare system is designed to protect us against major medical bills in later years, it only provides for care at home under certain specified and very strict conditions. The cost of these services can greatly impact personal savings, lifestyles, and in some cases, limits financial independence as a result of average care facilities running at between 40-80,000 dollars a year.

Divorce rates also have a significant impact in America today on the capacity of many women to produce long-term personal wealth. Despite divorce rates up to 50%, the result is a loss of income and often a dramatic change in the way women live. As the psychological impact of family separation, most divorced women are not used to their own finances, and many have little faith in their senior years ' position in financial planning.

Most divorced women often need to reintegrate into the workforce after years of unemployment to support or maintain existing living standards while still taking on primary care responsibilities. In this situation, women are, therefore, likely to have access to less capital, restricted years of retirement assets, and little experience in dealing with funding and risk management issues.

Failure to manage risk For many women, the way they deal with the inherent risks facing us all. The risk of premature death or disability in particular. This is particularly true when it concerns the principal household earner. To homemakers, the possibility of a financial loss is even greater, depending on the single income of a partner. While women are at greater risk in this case, quite often, there is not adequate insurance coverage to ensure a sufficient income replacement after primary years of rearing. Many couples focus more on the payment of college expenses than on retirement or loss of income. In fact, most people in this scenario do not take into account the number of years of female life expectancy in this calculation in terms of insurance coverage.

As a result of insufficient insurance coverage, many women are left without sufficient income to support their children. Many have to sell their homes and get their kids out of their neighborhood, schools, and friends. Typically, women in the situation now have to return to the workforce after many years of unemployment. It naturally leads to a shift in focus on immediate revenue needs, and pension issues frequently fall short of a priority.

In most situations, sufficient income substitution coverage is the result of poor guidance or other priorities. But many husbands are hesitant because of negative perceptions and outdated views to provide adequate coverage. In some societies, it is not uncommon for husbands to oppose the insurance idea altogether because they fear they would abandon the wealthy of their wives and provide future husbands with opportunities.

There is also evidence that some women are reluctant to rely on the safety of partners in spite of the recognized threats that they need. Women in this situation should understand how important insurance is in wealth creation and risk mitigation for families and women in particular. A properly placed insurance plan can often create an "instant property" and prevent unnecessary uncertainty and retirement plans from being sacrificed.

279

Although the number of women working in the workplace is high at all levels, women are less likely to work for retirement plan companies. When employer-sponsored plans are available to women, they appear to be more cautious investors and often do not fully understand how to optimize their investment plan choices. No access to retirement plans funded by employers; women risk becoming more dependent on social services, for example, Social Security and Medicare, to provide pension funds.

Over the years, the Social Security system has provided millions of elderly America ns with additional income, the social security system's lengthy-term financial viability is now in question. Unless the US Congress lacks the political will to intervene and change the current system, the Social Security System is scheduled to cease paying the current benefits in full by 2041. About 78 percent of currently scheduled payments are expected to be paid at that time. This will have an enormous impact on millions of veterans of Generation X and married women who match their demographic generation.

The personal savings rate of America ns is another significant issue for women. America 's personal savings rates fell for years until the current economic crisis in 2009. In 2005, this country's saving rates dropped into negative territory. It means that America ns spent more money than they won. Since the Great Depression, this saving rate has not been seen, when the nation experienced thousands of business failures and job losses. A lower savings rate is partially due to the increase in the value of other assets such as shares, bonds, and real estate in America over recent years. However, exposure to low-interest rates often discourages savings and encourages lending for big-ticket items such as vehicles and personal property.

In reality, our economy is now consumed. In all economic circumstances, government and media are encouraged to spend record amounts on further stimulating our economy. Although higher spending rates are good for the US economy, this is risky behavior for America 's retirement planning. "Americans feel like it's wimpy to save," David Wyss, chief economist at Standard & Poor's New York City, said. "The idea is to put away old-age money, and we just don't." There is actually no proof that women save at better prices than men in America.

Creating a sound financial future has never been an easy task for the vast majority of working people in America. The job with the current state of the America n economy is now more complicated than ever. The 2008-09 economic downturn further exacerbates an already dynamic and daunting undertaking. The current economic crisis has given about wide-ranging loss of jobs, a deterioration of retirement plans, increasing inflation, budget deficits, and higher tax potential. It has and will continue to have a devastating impact on millions of America n families in the foreseeable future.

Americans, aiming to produce retirement savings, should be aware of the specific circumstances that make their path to financial independence more difficult and distinct from other America n nations. Women in this country today have more career opportunities and gains in income equality with men than ever before. Despite these progressions, women have to bear the additional burden of longer lifetimes, high divorce rates, and lower savings rates. It brings even more pressure on women to create a retirement portfolio to make sure their investments are not depleted, and the chances of financial security are decreased.

For many women, the good news is that many financial solutions are available to help them face their unique challenges and allow them to build and preserve their wealth. Therefore, as women get better educated and economically informed, they understand that they don't have to go alone. More women look for the advice of professional financial planners who can help them achieve their pension goals, tailor a financial status that fulfills their individual needs, and ensure financial security.

What A Living Positively can contribute to your Wellbeing

We are learning a great deal today about Divine Order, The Code, the Law of Attraction, and the like. If this were real, then we would definitely all benefit from learning how to live our lives a little better. And even if it is not real-what, must we risk by at least being a little more optimistic in our everyday lives? Our lives would definitely be more fun if we lived like that. Here are a few practical tips and hints to help you live your life more positive and up-to-date.

Try to spread a little love wherever you can. A kind word thought or action goes a long way. Do you think of a time when someone else said, or did you feel good, or something positive happened to Vous? Try to make someone else happier if you want to be yourself. Swap what you have with someone else if you want to be more plentiful.

Feeling thankful is one of the most important things you can do to help you live better. Even in the worst situations, one should always be grateful. I find it helps to maintain a journal of' Gratitude.' This is just a list of things for which I am grateful. I must be grateful for many things, and the very act of writing the list reminds me of them and makes me more hopeful. If you try, at first you may find it difficult to think about anything, but as you continue and keep to it, you will soon find it difficult to stop! Try to write it as you go along too. See if you can't think of five new things every day to add to it.

Affirmations are a strong way to help you still remain positive. Use them as often as possible. Make sure they are all positive, tense, and personal, though, and say to them what you want, not what you want. Write them down or tell them to yourself, in your mind or loudly, over and over until they become part of you. And if you look for evidence continuously that your arguments work, you will soon see a difference.

Read more to relax. Every day, a few minutes of relaxation will help you keep up. One good way to relax is to find a quiet place to stay, sit, or lie comfortably and concentrate your breathing for a while. A good way to relax, try saying' I am' in-breath and' in love' on the breath to stop the mind from wandering. Breathing in-I am.' Breathing in. Breathing out-' at peace." at peace.' I use this technique in my therapy groups, and it helps to really stop the mind from talking and relaxing. You only have to do this about ten minutes a day, and will benefit a lot, not least because you start to look forward to it and feel more in control of yourself and your life.

285

Watch your words! Watch your words! It is shocking that in one day, we can make several negative statements. And we can soon realize things we say if we repeat them often enough. One exercise that I find helpful is to watch on the phone what you think. Often, when someone moans at the other end, we quite simply agree without even knowing that we are doing it. Or you may have a friend who's a little moaner, and you just say' Yeah, yeah' to save yourself from the trouble to think of the answer. When you catch yourself, try to see if there is some way to make things more optimistic.

Think about what you really want in life. If, in every way, your life was great, how would it be? Write a paragraph or two that portrays your ideal life as though it had been. At least in this way, you know what you are striving for, and you can focus on it. Many positive people have a goal to aspire for and look forward to something when their goal has been accomplished. Mental scanning can also motivate us to be more optimistic. Build an image of yourself that looks best and lives your ideal life. Then make it a habit to think about it regularly, particularly early and late in the day. All right, so perhaps you aren't living your ideal life right now, but something you're not striving to is it?

Enable yourself to spend time reading books every day, watching movies, or games. You don't have to be' motivational' necessarily. Just those that you like and feel comfortable reading or watching. Seek not to read newspapers that contain bad news or watch television news. This will only motivate you to' prove' that the world is in a bad way. If something really important happens, you can hear it anyway.

Try and make a match by finding things good. "It's raining, of course, but never mind that the garden gets watered." Okay, so it's a bit of a' Pollyanna ' theme, but why not? It's going to make you feel better, and that's all about it, after all.

Above all, treat yourself well. Give yourself a little time to relax every day, drink plenty of water, and have the best and freshest food you can find. As a consequence, you will feel much better. And allow yourself to treat yourself occasionally. A small bar of chocolate or cream cake won't harm you (not allergic to them, of course). And then you must have something that you can appreciate. So spend time doing the things you want. You (and your work) would benefit from this much more.

Treat yourself as if you were a best friend of your own. You deserve it, after all.

Note, when you give yourself first, you can't give. Give yourself the good things in your life and spread them all around. And if people ask what they are getting, just say "a good dose of positiveness!"

Living With Family Members Without Hating One another

Times are tough in front of it.

Families were financially closer than ever.

Will you encourage yourself to stay at home?

Are you a boomer or maker of sandwiches who wonder how to take care of / pay your kids, parents, and saves on your retirement? Are you widowed or retired recently and wondering how you are going to achieve ends?

288

There are many reasons why staying with the family or caring for the family is a great option. When you live with loved ones, you prefer being with, or close to home, You seem to get better attention from parents and mates near and cheaper.

It is no wonder that 80% of the elderly population depends on family care.

It could just be a requirement in today's fragile economy.

You might be the kind of person who wants to stay in your own home or with someone you love instead of moving to a nursing facility. Care costs are also enormous. Even with medications and drugs, a lot of secret and unexpected expenses also remain without considering the challenge of finding a treatment center where patients and workers can appreciate and provide the care you need and deserve.

The strained economy hits everybody, especially the elderly who need their medication and still get their doctoral appointments to pay higher electricity costs. This is not a luxury. The cost of a nursing home is staggering, and my insurance and medication are not all covered. On average, operating expenses for a day and daycare facility vary from about $450.-700.00 per day. A day. A day.

But it might not be desirable to move in with your adult children.

Many people want to stay as long as possible alone.

How do you stay at home?

Prepare at an early stage. Take long-term care, but make sure you come with a reputable company that will be in business for years to come and respect its contracts.

Remember the community, driving range, physicians, care facilities, and the senior services when you buy what you think is your last home. When you can't drive, can you stay there? Can you use a local bus or taxis? Is your first floor home/bedroom? Could you handle the house and yard maintenance? Plan, schedule, schedule.

Purchase land and build a smaller house or garage for a caregiver or family member. It's an asset that you will hold, and if or if you need to sell, your property value will only increase.

Suggest renting a room to another senior and dividing other care costs home or home to make a garage or a cabin to A spouse or younger person's rent. You may even consider renting in return for university programs, divorcees, other citizens, as well as nuns or nephews beginning their lives.

Build an apartment onto your home, or if you move into the home of your children, build it so that they can remain confidential and come and go as you like.

With time going on, find a small group home run by a provider that normally takes 4-8 people only; charges are lower although they can do less for you medically, so consider your wellbeing and medical needs when choosing How to live with family members without having to hate. Make sure that you can sit down and do that knowing that, in exchange, you will be heard and respected and do the same thing.

If you have young adults or university adults, try not to criticize or comment on all aspects of their lives. They have to make their own mistakes-they have to learn from them. Let them know you are there, and you'll be happy to hear or give advice if they inquire. They have to make their own mistakes-they have to learn from them. Let them know you are there, and you'll be happy to hear or give advice if they inquire.
Try not to hang up on your way all the way. Get to compromise. Learn to compromise. It's all right if someone buys a laundry detergent other than you're used to. Choose your sides and do as little as possible.
Try not to hang up on your way all the way. Get to compromise. Learn to compromise. It's all right if someone buys a laundry detergent other than you're used to. Choose your sides and do as little as possible.

Know that there will be a honeymoon and a time of disillusionment if you wonder if you made the right decision, but that it will happen too.

It is inevitable to acknowledge the transition. Don't pin what was once the now and choose to find the good every day.

Allow each other to knock and be considerate for food, rest, and time alone.

Be sensitive— if your loved one behaves strange, it could go through something he couldn't express or verbalize — there's a time for delicate patience.

Schedule any meals or hours, but don't overdo it.

Do not expect your parents to do everything to care for you or chore support.

Find and offer ways to be desired. Enable us to work consistently.

293

Seek not to worry about your health or living conditions-maybe, not all is good, but it could still be better than your other options.

Do not reflect on your life options— such as dressing, going to church (or not), listening to the state of your marriage-doing more than therapy.

Make friends and friendships, don't expect your parents to be all yours.

Smile, be easy to come along, and give thanks— it is infectious, so perhaps you will get some in exchange.

Don't let it fester if you have a question. Sit down, say peace, talk about a possible solution, and let go of it. Of six months to a year after you get together, you'll start to settle down, but this is when the honeymoon starts to wear off— with the intention of getting away from that first time of disappointment. It takes up to two years to feel like home. Sometimes you may feel lonely, confused, and unknown.

Be sure to reach a club, a senior citizen center, or church-making new friends in your new community-even if it is difficult and scary. It will be worth it. We all need family. They all need friends.

Elders recognize your place of honor and dignity-you have a special place in your family, but before anyone else, you must realize and own that first. Incarnate a sense of understanding, trust, and respect within yourself, and other people begin to feel it when they are around you.

Expect you will have a big fight or misunderstanding at some point. Families do such things. It's all right. Forgive each other. Forgive each other. Be quick to say, "I'm so sorry." Even if crying and pouting are involved, so what? People often act crazy. What else could you do other than your family?

Love for the parents is part of who we are. No cash can purchase love. If you are truly fortunate to have a courageous

295

family that will be determined in one way to love and care for each other, please be thankful.

It's all right to be angry, hurt, or upset with a member of the family. Families are robust. You should love intensely and forgive quickly (or finally, in some cases). As Cheryl Kaye Tardif, my friend and fellow writer, says, "It is not about how to live with your family without heating them. It is about living with your family without killing them! You may hate all that you want." Family devotion is deep.

Life does not change, and people are not fine, but the family is wonderful.

Step 5--Link your passions to your target. Note that it is not enough to make a general-purpose relevant. You must also determine what tool you are going to use for this reason. Our goal could be to help others, but our approaches could be very different. Simply evaluate your list of interests and core competencies to learn how you can use them in your life to achieve your goal.

Step 6--Build a Statement of Purpose. Your personal statement is a concise statement as to why you are here in this world. It consists of two parts: a general objective and a method. Keep your statement of purpose as concise as possible and limited to just two sentences. Your first statement is what you want to do with your life–the legacy in Step 3. The second sentence is how you intend to achieve this–your method. My personal statement has always been to help as many people as I can realize their personal dreams. I achieve this by writing, coaching, and teaching others how to maximize their potential.

CONCLUSION

Dedicate Every day to Your Purpose Once you have defined and explained what your purpose is, you must dedicate yourself to this path. This can be easily achieved by doing something every day that pushes you toward your target. While those acts are small, if each day you do at least one thing which gets you closer to your goal, then by the end of the year that is 365 small steps. You will have taken 10,950 moves towards your main purpose by the end of 30 years. No matter how small those steps are, they will add up as time advances–so start today! When going to sleep at the end of each day, ask yourself if you have given yourself everything that you had to give that day.

Create a mindset never give up the path to your destination is never an easy one. Inevitably, you will face challenges, some minor, some very rising. Regardless of the challenges you face, it is crucial that you cultivate the courage to do whatever it takes to achieve your ultimate goals in life. Adversity will test

your resolve, and it is up to you to lift the sword and battle
every obstacle.

www.ingramcontent.com/pod-product-compliance
Lightning Source LLC
Chambersburg PA
CBHW031052250726
48655CB00004B/1399